Medical Management of Glaucoma

Second Edition

James C. Tsai, MD

Associate Professor of Ophthalmology
Director, Glaucoma Division
Homer McK. Rees Scholar
The Edward S. Harkness Eye Institute
Columbia University College of
Physicians and Surgeons

Max Forbes, MD

Professor Emeritus of Clinical Ophthalmology
The Edward S. Harkness Eye Institute
Columbia University College of
Physicians and Surgeons

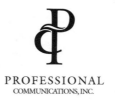

PROFESSIONAL
COMMUNICATIONS, INC.

Professional Communications, Inc.

A Medical Publishing Company

Marketing Office:
400 Center Bay Drive
West Islip, NY 11795
(t) 631/661-2852
(f) 631/661-2167

Editorial Office:
PO Box 10
Caddo, OK 74729-0010
(t) 580/367-9838
(f) 580/367-9989

For orders only, please call
1-800-337-9838

or visit our website at
www.pcibooks.com

ISBN: 1-884735-97-5

Printed in the United States of America

DISCLAIMER

The opinions expressed in this publication reflect those of the authors. However, the authors make no warranty regarding the contents of the publication. The protocols described herein are general and may not apply to a specific patient. Any product mentioned in this publication should be taken in accordance with the prescribing information provided by the manufacturer.

This text is printed on recycled paper.

DEDICATION

To our families for their love and support…

James C. Tsai

Tracey, Jessica, and Emily-Anne Tsai

Hsien Wang Tsai

David and Janet Tsai

Ming and Alison Tsai

Max Forbes

Avonell Marie Forbes

Brian, Julie, and Diane Forbes

ACKNOWLEDGMENT

To our patients, who continually inspire and challenge us to strive for better treatments for glaucoma. To Joel Legunn and Phyllis Freeny, for their assistance in the preparation of this manuscript. And to our chairman, Dr. Stanley Chang, for his encouragement and support.

TABLE OF CONTENTS

TABLES

FIGURES

1

Introduction: Primary
Open-Angle Glaucoma

The majority of patients diagnosed with open-angle glaucoma (OAG) present as adults with:
- Normal-appearing anterior segments
- Open angles
- An absence of secondary causes.

Primary open-angle glaucoma (POAG) is diagnosed when a patient has elevated intraocular pressure (IOP) and glaucomatous optic neuropathy (GON). Ocular hypertension (OH) is diagnosed when IOP is elevated and the optic nerve appears normal. Normal-pressure glaucoma (NPG) or normal-tension glaucoma (NTG) is diagnosed when the patient has normal pressures (confirmed by diurnal IOP testing) and GON. NTG has been noted to occur in approximately 25% to 40% of individuals diagnosed with OAG in population-based studies.[1-3] Finally, patients with consistently normal IOPs and suspicious-appearing optic nerves are diagnosed as NPG suspects.

Although elevated IOP may play a significant role in the pathogenesis of glaucoma and lowering of IOP is the only proven treatment, the definition of glaucoma has evolved from a disease caused by increased IOP to one characterized by an IOP-sensitive optic neuropathy.[4] In the most recent edition of the American Academy of Ophthalmology's Preferred Practice Pattern, POAG is defined as *a multifactorial optic neuropathy in which there is a characteristic acquired loss of retinal ganglion cells (RGC) and atrophy of the optic nerve.*[5]

The multifactorial nature of glaucoma is illustrated by the far-ranging spectrum of patients with garden-variety POAG to those with NTG. In addition to the risk factor of elevated IOP, there is mounting evidence that insufficient blood flow to the optic nerve head is also a contributing factor in the pathogenesis of glaucoma.[6] It has also been postulated that the presence of excitotoxins, stimulated by excessive release of glutamate, results in RGC death and that neuroprotection may be a viable strategy in the treatment of GON.[7]

Characteristics of POAG

Major characteristics of POAG include:
- Presence of progressive optic nerve damage (**Table 1.1**)
- Adult onset
- Open normal-appearing anterior chamber angles
- Absence of other explanations for progressive GON, such as elevated IOP due to pigment dispersion or pseudoexfoliation.[5]

It is also important to note that POAG represents a spectrum of diseases and that susceptibility to damage of the optic nerve in these diseases demonstrates interpatient variability.[5] The following chapters will discuss the diagnosis, epidemiology, etiology, progression, and treatment of POAG.

TABLE 1.1 — EVIDENCE OF PROGRESSIVE OPTIC NERVE DAMAGE

Optic Disc or Retinal Nerve Fiber Layer
- Diffuse or focal narrowing or notching of disc rim (especially at the inferior or superior poles)
- Diffuse or localized abnormalities of the retinal nerve fiber layer (especially at the inferior or superior poles)
- Nerve fiber layer hemorrhage(s)
- Asymmetric appearance of the optic disc rim between fellow eyes (suggesting loss of neural tissue)

Abnormalities in Visual Field*
- Nasal step or scotoma
- Inferior or superior actuate scotoma
- Paracentral scotoma
- Generalized depression
- Persistent worsening of the correct-pattern standard deviation (CPSD) on automated threshold perimetry

* In the absence of other explanations for a field defect.

American Academy of Ophthalmology Preferred Practice Patterns Committee Glaucoma Panel. *Preferred Practice Patterns. Primary Open-Angle Glaucoma.* San Francisco, Calif: American Academy of Ophthalmology; 2000:1-38.

REFERENCES

1.   Werner EB. Normal-tension glaucoma. In: Ritch R, Shields MB, Krupin T, eds. *The Glaucomas*. 2nd ed. St. Louis, Mo: Mosby; 1996:781.

2.   Klein BE, Klein R, Sponsel WE, et al. Prevalence of glaucoma. The Beaver Dam Eye Study. *Ophthalmology*. 1992;99:1499-1504.

3.   Dielemans I, Vingerling JR, Wolfs RC, Hofman A, Grobbee DE, de Jong PT. The prevalence of primary open-angle glaucoma in a population-based study in The Netherlands. The Rotterdam Study. *Ophthalmology*. 1994;101:1851-1855.

4.   Lichter PR. Expectations from clinical trials: results of the Early Manifest Glaucoma Trial. *Arch Ophthalmol*. 2002;120:1371-1372.

5.   American Academy of Ophthalmology Preferred Practice Patterns Committee Glaucoma Panel. *Preferred Practice Patterns. Primary Open-Angle Glaucoma*. San Francisco, Calif: American Academy of Ophthalmology; 2000:1-38.

6.   Hayreh SS. Factors influencing blood flow in the optic nerve head. *J Glaucoma*. 1997;6:412-425.

7.   Levin LA. Relevance of the site of injury of glaucoma to neuroprotective strategies. *Surv Ophthalmol*. 2001;45(suppl):S243-S249.

2

Patient Assessment: Ocular History and Exam

An accurate diagnosis of a patient presenting with signs and symptoms of glaucoma requires a comprehensive evaluation, including:

- Ocular, medical (including medication), and family histories
- A complete review of symptoms
- A complete ocular examination.

Ocular History

The ocular history includes assessment of the extent, duration, severity, and interval history of current and past symptoms experienced by the patient. However, in the majority of cases, primary open-angle glaucoma (POAG) has few detectable symptoms until considerable vision loss and/or visual field defects have occurred. All prior anti-glaucoma therapy, including medications, laser, and surgery, should be noted in detail.

■ Blurred Vision and Ocular Pain

Blurring of vision, with and without halos, has a number of causes, and is not usually associated with POAG unless there is rapid change of intraocular pressure (IOP) and/or extreme elevations in IOP. Ocular pain is infrequent in glaucoma because of the eye's compensatory mechanisms to elevated IOP. However, when elevation of IOP is rapid or sustained IOP elevation is very high (eg, in the range of 50 mm Hg), patients may experience pain around the globe accompanied by nausea and vomiting.[1]

- **Patient-Reported Visual Field Defects and Loss of Visual Acuity**

Visual field defects that accompany chronic POAG usually consist of mid-peripheral visual field loss. As such, this loss is usually undetected by most patients until the disease is well advanced. However, in normal-tension glaucoma (NTG) and in POAG associated with myopia, patients may become aware of early visual field defects that occur close to fixation.[2] Optic atrophy accompanied by visual acuity loss may be seen in certain forms of open-angle glaucoma (OAG), even without the characteristic disc cupping noted in chronic glaucoma. When a patient reports loss of visual acuity (especially in the setting of advanced glaucomatous field loss just above or below central fixation), aggressive therapeutic measures to further lower IOP are clearly indicated.[2]

Medical History

- **Systemic Disease**

A number of systemic diseases may be risk factors for the development of OAG, but these associations have not been clearly demonstrated. For example, a relationship between systemic hypertension and POAG may exist. Elevated blood pressure (BP) has been associated with increases in IOP, and some studies have shown an association between systemic hypertension and POAG.[3-5] In contrast, low vascular perfusion pressure has also been associated with an increased prevalence of POAG. It has been hypothesized that a dramatic decline in BP overnight may result in low vascular perfusion pressure and thus diminished optic nerve perfusion. Of note, significant decreases in nocturnal BP have been shown to produce an increased risk for the development of POAG and normal-pressure glaucoma (NPG).[6,7] Finally, diabetes mellitus has been reported to be a risk factor for POAG in hospital-based studies, although the associated risk may be overestimated due to the increased prevalence of patients with diabetes in these studies. Population-based studies, on the other hand, do not support a clear association of diabetes mellitus and the occurrence of POAG.[5]

■ Systemic Medications

It is important to determine the presence or history of respiratory allergies, asthma, or other causes of dyspnea in patients being treated for POAG. These patients may be at risk for the onset or exacerbation of bronchospasm with respiratory insufficiency when treated for glaucoma with β-blockers. Conversely, systemic medications used to treat these respiratory conditions may induce the onset of glaucoma or exacerbate a pre-existing glaucoma.

Medications with anticholinergic or atropinelike effects may precipitate angle-closure glaucoma in patients with anatomically narrow angles.[1] Intensive use of topical or systemic corticosteroids may elevate IOP within 1 to 2 weeks, but the pressure elevation is usually reversed within days to weeks of terminating treatment. On the other hand, patients on chronic low-dose steroid therapy may not develop elevated IOP for months, thereby making the diagnosis more difficult and mandating careful monitoring in such cases. Corticosteroid-induced elevations in IOP lead to an OAG that closely resembles POAG. In summary, it is important to determine if patients presenting with elevated IOP are currently being treated with corticosteroids, and if patients with GON and normal IOP were treated previously with corticosteroids.[8]

Family History

Genetics are known to play a significant role in the onset of glaucoma. Therefore, a family history of

OAG might predispose an individual to developing the disease. An estimated 13% to 47% of POAG cases are familial; there is also a 5- to 20-fold greater prevalence rate of POAG among patients with a family history.[5] In the presence of a positive family history of glaucoma, patients should be observed more carefully, especially those with ocular hypertension (OH).

Visual Acuity Measurement

In patients with OAG, additional visual information (eg, spatial resolution) may be obtained by utilizing low-contrast and low-luminance stimuli, with or without different stimulus shapes. In addition, various visual field locations may be tested, such as the paracentral region, in which visual field loss often occurs first. Visual acuity tests have been developed that use low-contrast visual stimuli for possible detection of adverse effects of glaucoma under conditions of low visibility.[9]

Intraocular Pressure

■ Normal, Borderline, and Abnormal IOP

Large-scale population studies have demonstrated that the mean IOP for the general population is approximately 15.5 mm Hg. Moreover, two standard deviations on either side of this mean value have been agreed upon to define the boundaries of the normal IOP range—10 mm Hg to 21 mm Hg.[10] The difficulty inherent in defining a normal IOP range for a particular individual—especially with regard to the onset of glaucoma—lies in the variable susceptibility to damage from different ranges of eye pressure. Many patients do not develop glaucomatous optic neuropathy (GON) at IOPs >21 mm Hg, whereas others may demonstrate progressive field loss at IOPs significantly <21 mm Hg.[10] The graphic distribution for these popu-

18

lations resembles a Gaussian curve skewed slightly toward higher pressures. In one major population-based study, this shift in the Gaussian distribution was postulated to represent two populations—a large normal group and a smaller group representing those with unrecognized glaucoma. A proposed distribution for two such groups is shown in **Figure 2.1**.[11] This example illustrates that the defining borders between normal and abnormal IOPs overlap and are not well defined.

■ Methods of Tonometry

In the clinical setting, IOP is determined by measuring the force necessary to indent or flatten (applanate) the surface of the eye. There are two common methods for conducting these measurements:

- Schiotz, or indentation, tonometry
- Applanation tonometry, which measures the force required to flatten the cornea.

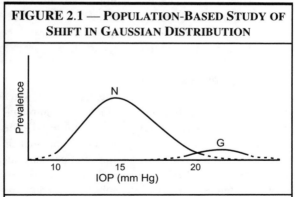

FIGURE 2.1 — POPULATION-BASED STUDY OF SHIFT IN GAUSSIAN DISTRIBUTION

Theoretical distribution of intraocular pressures (IOPs) in nonglaucoma (N) and glaucoma (G) populations, showing overlap between the two groups (dotted lines represent uncertainty of extreme values in both populations).

Shields MB. *Textbook of Glaucoma*. 4th ed. Baltimore, Md: Williams and Wilkins; 1998:47.

Schiotz Tonometry

Schiotz tonometry, the older of the two methods, measures the depth of indentation of the cornea by a known weight that is applied with the patient supine. The depth of indentation, shown by a scale on the tonometer, is converted by means of a special table to a corresponding IOP reading in millimeters of mercury.[11,12] The advantages of the Schiotz tonometer are its:

- Portability
- Ease of use
- Low cost.

However, its accuracy of measurement is limited by:

- Variations in corneal curvature
- Rigidity and volume of the eye, which determine the influence of the weight itself on IOP.

In addition, the precision of readings may be affected by incorrect technique and/or calibration of the scale, although some of these inaccuracies have been addressed by the newer electronic devices.[13] Schiotz tonometry is rarely used in clinical practice.

Applanation Tonometry

Applanation tonometry is currently the gold standard for measuring IOP, and the Goldmann applanation tonometer—mounted on a slit lamp—is the standard instrument for this procedure. Applanation tonometry is based on the principle that pressure inside a dry, thin-walled sphere equals the force necessary to flatten the surface of the sphere divided by the area flattened. For the Goldmann applanation tonometer, the applanating force measured is that required to flatten an area of the cornea 3.06 mm in diameter.[13] This diameter has been derived to cancel the opposing effects of tear film surface tension on the tonometer and resistance of the cornea to deformation. The influence of ocular rigidity is virtually eliminated as a source of error because the volume of fluid displacement is minimal. The force required to applanate is accurately determined by means of a split-field prism that divides the circular meniscus of the tear film which represents the flattened area of the cornea into semicircles. When the margins of the semicircles overlap, an area of the cornea 3.06 mm in diameter is flattened. The IOP in millimeters of mercury is equal to 10 times the flattening force (in grams). This technique is safe, simple to perform, and highly accurate.[11-13] Errors can occur with the Goldmann tonometer due to:

- Misalignment of the semicircles of the meniscus
- Misjudgment of the width of the meniscus
- Breath-holding or Valsalva's maneuver
- Squeezing of the eyelids
- Finger pressure on the globe by the examiner
- Inaccurate calibration of the device.

In addition, corneal thickness (to be discussed later) can have a significant impact on the accuracy of the IOP readings.

Other Tonometry Devices

The Perkins applanation tonometer is essentially a portable version of the Goldmann tonometer. It utilizes the same biprism split-field arrangement, its light source is battery powered, and a counterbalance allows it to be used in the vertical or horizontal position— when the patient is either sitting or lying down. It is particularly useful for measuring IOP in infants under general anesthesia, children who are not comfortable sitting at the slit lamp, and for patients who tend to hold their breath while at the slit lamp, a situation that affects IOP.[12]

The pneumatic tonometer (pneumatonometer) measures IOP by means of a sensor, consisting of a gas-inflated chamber covered by an elastic membrane, that applanates the cornea. Air pressure in the chamber, which rises rapidly before falling to a trough at applanation, is then converted by a transducer to a digital reading of IOP. This device is especially valuable for measuring IOP after corneal transplantation and in eyes with corneal scarring, edema, or other irregularity.[11-13]

The Tonopen is a hand-held device that utilizes a pressure transducer (in accordance with the principle of Mackay-Marg tonometry) to measure the pressure applied via a plunger to flatten a small area of cornea (1.5 mm diameter). That measurement is equal to the IOP at the instant when corneal resistance to distortion is transferred from the plunger to a surrounding sleeve. IOP is displayed digitally. Several measurements are made on each eye. This portable device is useful for measuring IOP in corneas with known irregularities and can easily be used by technicians and other nonphysicians. Major drawbacks include its overestimation of IOP in the lower pressure ranges and underestimation of IOP in the much higher pressure ranges.[11,12]

A variation of the Goldmann tonometer is the noncontact, or air-puff, tonometer. This instrument does not measure force or pressure directly. By means of an optical detector, it measures the time necessary for a jet of air of increasing force to flatten the cornea; longer time is equivalent to greater force and therefore higher IOP. Measured time in milliseconds was calibrated to IOP by means of corresponding Goldmann tonometer measurements. In practice, noncontact tonometer readings compare favorably in accuracy to those of the Goldmann tonometer, except at the higher ranges of IOP. A major advantage is the avoidance of contact between cornea and instrument, thereby eliminating the risk of infection.[13]

■ Central Corneal Thickness

The Ocular Hypertension Treatment Study (OHTS), among others, concluded that central corneal thickness (CCT) has a significant effect on IOP readings.[14] For corneas thicker than 600 microns, IOP may be overestimated by applanation tonometry. In contrast, for corneas thinner than 500 microns, IOP may be significantly higher than that obtained by applanation.[15]

In a study of IOP using manometric methods, Ehler and colleagues found that 44% of NTG eyes would have to be reclassified as having POAG, whereas 35% of ocular hypertension eyes would have to be reclassified as normal.[16] African Americans appear to have significantly thinner CCT measurements than Caucasians, Asians, or Hispanics, thereby causing a substantial under-reading of true IOP.[17] In a retrospective study of the initial visit characteristics of consecutive patients with POAG presenting to a glaucoma specialist, multivariate analysis demonstrated that thinner CCT was significantly associated with greater perimetric mean deviation and Advanced Glaucoma Intervention Study (AGIS) visual field score, and increased vertical and horizontal cup-disc ratios.[18] Moreover, CCT was a consistent and powerful predictor of the extent of glaucomatous damage in these patients.

From the aforementioned studies, we can conclude that the accuracy of baseline IOP levels (prior to treatment) is in doubt without CCT measurements. Under these circumstances, it is possible that a sizable number of patients may be either undertreated or overtreated based on artifacts introduced into applanation IOP readings by variations in CCT. These data suggest strongly that corneal pachymetry should be performed routinely to determine CCT in patients suspected of having glaucoma whether IOP is elevated or normal.[19]

■ Diurnal Variation of IOP

A single measurement of IOP (as part of the glaucoma examination) may not suffice to establish the presence or absence of elevated pressure, since IOP is subject to diurnal variation. In individuals without glaucoma, the normal variation is from 2 to 6 mm Hg. A diurnal variation >10 mm Hg is often indicative of glaucoma.[10,13] While many individuals experience peak IOPs in the morning, others reach peak pressures in the afternoon or evening. Moreover, in some patients, there may be no reproducible or discernible diurnal pattern.[13] Therefore, it may be necessary to measure IOP at various times throughout the day to detect this variation and establish a pattern of elevated IOP in an individual who is suspected of having glaucoma.

■ Corticosteroids

As noted earlier in the discussion of systemic medications, corticosteroids may induce secondary elevations in IOP. Patients should therefore be questioned during the examination about their use of systemic, nasal, or topical corticosteroids.

■ Other Factors Affecting IOP

Emotions, such as stress, have not been shown to have a significant effect on IOP in patients with POAG. However, stress, which may cause pupillary dilation, can induce acute angle-closure glaucoma (AACG) in susceptible individuals with narrow angles. Transient elevations in IOP in patients with glaucoma have been described following their consumption of very large volumes of water (beyond what is normally consumed on a daily basis). Excessive intake of caffeine by patients with POAG may also induce elevations in IOP, but this phenomenon is not well understood. It may be of value, however, to caution POAG patients with poorly controlled IOPs to limit caffeine intake.[1]

■ Slit-Lamp Examination

The slit lamp should be used to determine the existence of or to rule out abnormalities in various ocular structures. With a slit-lamp examination, baseline observations are used for future reference in evaluating the potential progression of the glaucoma condition. **Table 2.1** outlines some of the areas that should receive attention during the slit-lamp exam.

Gonioscopy

Gonioscopy, a clinical method of examining the structures of the anterior chamber angle, is a fundamental technique used to diagnose an individual's type of glaucoma. An accurate assessment of the chamber angle is necessary for determining the appropriate treatment, since therapies indicated for one type of glaucoma may be contraindicated in other glaucomas.[13]

The anterior chamber angle may be viewed either by direct or indirect gonioscopy. Direct gonioscopy involves using a Koeppe goniolens placed on the cornea and directly viewing the angle with separate light source (**Figure 2.2**). Indirect gonioscopy relies on a gonioprism, and the prototype is the Goldmann gonioprism, which has a single mirror to reflect light from the angle and requires rotation of the prism to view the entire angle (**Figure 2.3**). A four-mirror Zeiss lens eliminates the need to rotate the lens to obtain a 360° view of the angle. Indentation (or pressure) gonioscopy can be performed with the Zeiss lens because it is curved to fit directly against the cornea similar to a contact lens. The lens is indented manually across the cornea; the procedure serves to distinguish between appositional angle closure and peripheral anterior synechiae (PAS). Areas of appositional angle closure are reversible with indentation pressure, whereas synechiae are not.[20,21]

■ Grading Systems
A number of systems have been devised to grade angle width and assess the degree of or potential for angle closure. The Shaffer system describes the angu-

TABLE 2.1 — SLIT-LAMP EVALUATION

Ocular Structure	Possible Abnormalities
Cornea (epithelium and endothelium)	Edema, abnormal stromal thickness, Fuchs' corneal endothelial dystrophy, peripheral anterior synechiae associated with irido-corneal endothelial syndromes, pigment deposition on the corneal endothelium, keratic precipitates
Anterior chamber	Peripheral and axial anterior chamber depth to establish normal values and to rule out a narrow chamber; axial depth to determine position of lens and possible narrowing of angle; changes in axial anterior chamber depth that may be indicative of malignant glaucoma
Iris	Transpupillary iris transillumination to uncover peripupillary defects and pigmentary dispersion syndrome; evaluate texture of iris and determine presence of nevi or membranes
Lens	Exfoliation on anterior surface of lens; exfoliation or pigment on the zonules; pigment deposited between posterior lens surface, zonules, and hyaloid; all other lenticular opacities

Epstein DL. Examination of the eye. In: Epstein DL, Allingham RR, Schuman JS, eds. *Chandler and Grant's Glaucoma*. 4th ed. Baltimore, Md: Williams and Wilkins; 1997:33-40.

FIGURE 2.2 — DIRECT GONIOSCOPY

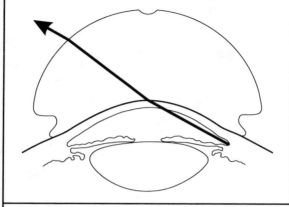

With direct gonioscopy, light from the angle is viewed directly through the Koeppe lens.

Kolker AE, Hetherington J, eds. *Becker-Shaffer's Diagnosis and Therapy of the Glaucomas.* 5th ed. St. Louis, Mo: CV Mosby Co; 1983.

lar width of the iridocorneal recess[20] and is the most frequently used classification system (**Table 2.2**). The more detailed Spaeth grading system adds a description of peripheral iris contour, presumed insertion of the iris root, and actual insertion of iris root as determined by indentation gonioscopy.[13]

■ **Clinical Findings**

In addition to evaluating for primary angle-closure glaucoma (PACG), gonioscopy should be performed to determine the presence of PAS and posttraumatic angle recession. It is also important to look for signs of neovascularization—normal vessels in the angle are oriented radially along the iris or circumferentially in the ciliary body face, as opposed to abnormal new vessels that cross the scleral spur. Although pigmentation of the trabecular meshwork is a

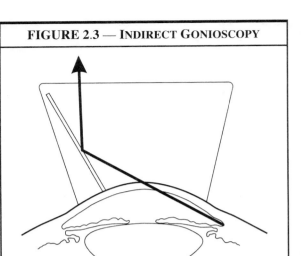

FIGURE 2.3 — INDIRECT GONIOSCOPY

Indirect gonioscopy relies on reflection of light by a mirror to observe the angle.

Kolker AE, Hetherington J, eds. *Becker-Shaffer's Diagnosis and Therapy of the Glaucomas*. 5th ed. St. Louis, Mo: CV Mosby Co; 1983.

normal occurrence with aging, heavy pigmentation, often a sign of pigment dispersion syndrome or pseudoexfoliation syndrome, should be noted.[13]

Optic Disc

The visible section of the optic nerve head is referred to as the optic disc. Its specific morphology provides visibly discernible clinical signs of glaucomatous changes. The optic disc is usually a slightly vertical oval, and it contains a central depression—the physiologic cup—a pale area partially or completely devoid of axons with exposure of the lamina cribrosa.[22] The nerve tissue between the cup and the disc margin is

TABLE 2.2 — SHAFFER CLASSIFICATION OF THE ANTERIOR CHAMBER ANGLE

Grade	Angle Width	Potential for Angle Closure
4	45° (wide open)	Improbable
3	20° to 45°	Unlikely
2	20°	Possible
1	10° (very narrow)	Probable
0 – Slit	Totally or partially closed	Present or very likely

American Academy of Ophthalmology. *Glaucoma. Basic and Clinical Science Course 2003-2004.* San Francisco, Calif: American Academy of Ophthalmology; 2003:30-38; AND Foster PJ, Johnson GJ. Primary angle closure: classification and clinical features. In: Hitchings RA, ed. *Glaucoma.* London: BMJ Publishing Group; 2000:145-152.

the neural rim, an important landmark in the ophthalmic investigation of the optic nerve.[13,24] The disc, cup, and neural rim display considerable inter-individual variations in shape and size, but the sizes of the disc and cup are related; for example, a large disc usually has a large cup.[22,23]

■ **Stereoscopic Slit-lamp Biomicroscopy**

There are several methods of examining the optic disc, including direct and indirect ophthalmoscopy. These techniques do not, however, detect many of the subtle changes in the disc or peripapillary area associated with glaucoma. Stereoscopic evaluation provides a more effective method of observing these minute glaucomatous changes in optic disc topography. The most effective method of stereoscopic viewing is with a slit lamp and either a Hruby lens, a posterior-pole contact lens, or a hand-held 90- or 78-diopter lens.[13,22] Stereoscopic photographs should be obtained to establish a baseline for later comparison of disease progression.

■ Evaluating Characteristics of the Cup

Comparing the diameter of the optic disc to that of the optic cup provides a marker for progression of glaucomatous optic nerve atrophy. Because of the vertical oval shape of the disc and the horizontally oriented oval shape of the cup, the horizontal cup/disc (C/D) ratio is usually larger than the vertical C/D ratio. However, the vertical C/D ratio increases faster than the horizontal C/D ratio in early and intermediate stages of glaucoma.[24] When determining this ratio, it is important to specify whether the cup is defined by a change in color or by a change in the contour between the central area of the disc and the surrounding rim, as well as which diameter (horizontal, vertical, or longest) of the disc is being measured. The most descriptive method is to specify the color and contour of the horizontal and vertical dimensions. Normal C/D ratios range from <0.3 (66% of normal individuals) to >0.5 (6% of normal individuals).[13]

A distinguishing factor between glaucomatous and nonglaucomatous optic neuropathy is that in the former, there is enlargement and deepening of the optic cup and a pronounced loss of the neural rim.[24] In addition, if there is focal or selective loss of the neural rim occurring in the inferior and/or superior pole of the disc, the cup itself becomes vertically elongated (**Figure 2.4**).[13] If optic atrophy continues to proceed, glaucomatous cupping of the disc becomes total with complete loss of the neural rim. The remaining structure is a white, pale optic disc with distortion of all vessels at the disc margin. Saucerization is an unusual form of glaucomatous cupping in which backward bowing or shallow cupping extends to the disc margin with no appreciable change in the dimensions of the central cup (**Figure 2.5**).

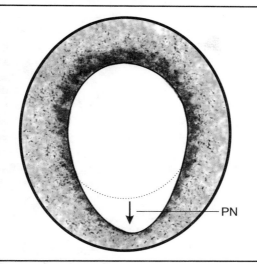

FIGURE 2.4 — GLAUCOMATOUS OPTIC ATROPHY

PN

Abbreviation: PN, polar notch.

Inferior enlargement of cup (arrow) compared with an original cup outline (dotted line) in glaucomatous optic atrophy.

Adapted from: Shields MB. *Textbook of Glaucoma*. 4th ed. Baltimore, Md: Williams and Wilkins; 1998:87.

■ Pallor

Enlargement of the optic cup may exceed the area of pallor in early glaucomatous optic atrophy. This may result in underestimation of the C/D ratio if the disc is evaluated by focusing solely on the area of pallor and overlooking the extent of cupping. The outermost border of cupping may be determined by noting the twisting of the disc vessels at the border of the cup. This divergence between the pallor and the cup is common and is an important indication of early glaucomatous cupping.[23]

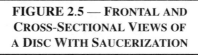

FIGURE 2.5 — FRONTAL AND CROSS-SECTIONAL VIEWS OF A DISC WITH SAUCERIZATION

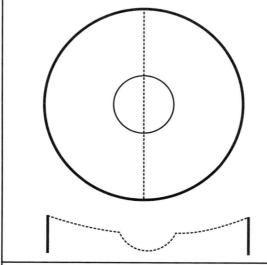

Epstein DL, ed. *Chandler and Grant's Glaucoma*. 4th ed. Baltimore, Md: Williams and Wilkins; 1997.

■ Peripapillary Changes

The optic disc may be encircled by zones of different widths, circumferences, and degrees of pigmentation. These include zone alpha, a peripapillary crescent comprised of increased pigmentation, and zone beta, a chorioscleral crescent that is often associated with thinning or absence of the choroid next to the disc.[23] When there is peripapillary chorioretinal atrophy associated with glaucoma, these two zones are larger and occur more often than in normal eyes. The alpha zone is also characterized by pigment irregularities in the retinal pigment epithelium. The beta zone signals complete loss of retinal pigment epithelium and a significantly reduced retinal photoreceptor count.[23]

■ **Optic Disc Hemorrhages**

Optic disc hemorrhages are often indicative of GON and occur as either splinter- or flame-shaped hemorrhages at the edges of the optic disc.[24] These hemorrhages rarely occur in normal eyes and are found in approximately 4% to 7% of glaucomatous eyes. Since disc hemorrhages occur in association with other optic nerve diseases, they are not a reliable diagnostic screening tool for glaucoma. However, in a patient with known OAG (especially in the setting of NPG), their presence is an important marker for impending glaucomatous progression and/or inconsistent or inadequate control of IOP. Disc hemorrhages also occur more frequently in patients with NPG than in patients with nonglaucomatous optic nerve cupping with known intracranial mass lesions.[25] Moreover, an increased frequency of disc hemorrhages during follow-up is associated with an increased risk of progression in patients with early manifest OAG.[26]

■ **Retinal Nerve Fiber Layer Defects**

The retinal nerve fibers and optic nerve head are comprised of axons that originate in the retinal ganglion cells, and optic atrophy in glaucoma is associated with loss of axons in the nerve fiber layer. Defects in the retinal nerve fiber layer (RNFL) usually precede detectable visual field loss.[27] Visible defects in the RNFL represent the loss of specific axon bundles, which eventually result in changes at the neural rim. Nerve bundle defects can be seen as distinct dark stripes (wedge-shaped aberrations in the peripapillary area) or loss of normal striations of the retina. These defects may represent the most important early sign of GON.[22]

■ **Optic Cup Diameter**

The sizes of the optic disc and optic cup are interrelated. That is to say, a large disc usually has a large cup. In contrast, a small disc has a small cup, and cupping may not occur at all. Therefore, it is possible to misdiagnose GON in a small disc with a small C/D ratio. Conversely, a large C/D ratio may not indicate the presence of glaucoma in the setting of a large optic disc size, especially if there is no other pathologic sign or morphologic change indicative of glaucomatous damage, such as a RNFL defect or neural rim loss.[28]

■ Asymmetry of Optic Disc Cupping

The extent of optic disc cupping is usually symmetric in normal eyes, and thus any asymmetry in the C/D ratio >0.2 may be considered an early sign of glaucoma. Early glaucoma should be considered even if the asymmetric larger cup appears to be physiologically normal in dimension. When physiologic cupping is symmetric, however, it is difficult to determine whether glaucoma is present, since there is marked interindividual variability in cup size.[22,28]

■ The Myopic Optic Disc

Because of its sloping and/or tilted contour, the myopic eye presents unique obstacles for proper assessment of the optic disc. Therefore, difficulties arise in correctly evaluating the neural disc rim in the myopic eye. Due to the tilted shape, portions of the disc rim may appear to be thinner than normal, thereby suggesting a pathologic condition. Moreover, the size of the disc and depth of the cup may be misinterpreted in a highly myopic eye.[22,28]

Systemic Evaluation

In addition to the above-noted ophthalmic evaluation, a problem-focused systemic evaluation should also be undertaken. For example, where indicated in the diagnostic workup of NPG, this may include determination of blood pressure and/or heart rate, carotid artery examination to rule out bruits, and neurologic evaluation. Particular attention should also be directed to the effects of both current and previous systemic medications, including corticosteroids.

2

REFERENCES

1. Epstein DL. The patient's history: symptoms of glaucoma. In: Epstein DL, Allingham RR, Schuman JS, eds. *Chandler and Grant's Glaucoma*. 4th ed. Baltimore, Md: Williams and Wilkins; 1997:25-32.

2. Hitchings R. Normal-tension glaucoma. In: Yanoff M, Duker JS, eds. *Ophthalmology*. London: Mosby; 1999:12.12.1-4.

3. Dielemans I, Vingerling JR, Algra D, Hofman A, Grobbee DE, de Jong PT. Primary open-angle glaucoma, intraocular pressure, and systemic blood pressure in the general elderly population. The Rotterdam Study. *Ophthalmology*. 1995; 102:54-60.

4. Wilson MR, Hertzmark E, Walker AM, Childs-Shaw K, Epstein DL. A case-controlled study of risk factors in open angle glaucoma. *Arch Ophthalmol*. 1987;105:1066-1071.

5. Fraser SG. Epidemiology of primary open angle glaucoma. In: Hitchings RA, ed. *Glaucoma*. London: BMJ Publishing Group; 2000:9-15.

6. Tielsch JM, Katz J, Sommer A, Quigley HA, Javitt JC. Hypertension, perfusion pressure, and primary open-angle glaucoma. A population-based assessment. *Arch Ophthalmol*. 1995;113:216-221.

7. Meyer JH, Brandi-Dohan J, Funk J. Twenty four hour blood pressure monitoring in normal tension glaucoma. *Br J Ophthalmol*. 1996;80:864-867.

8. Johnson DH. Corticosteroid glaucoma. In: Epstein DL, Allingham RR, Schuman JS, eds. *Chandler and Grant's Glaucoma*. 4th ed. Baltimore, Md: Williams and Wilkins; 1997:404-411.

9. Breton ME, Drum BA. Functional testing in glaucoma: Visual psychophysics and electrophysiology. In: Ritch R, Shields MB, Krupin T, eds. *The Glaucomas*. 2nd ed. St. Louis, Mo: Mosby; 1996:677-699.

10. Tsai JC. Intraocular pressure. In: Hitchings RA, ed. *Glaucoma*. London: BMJ Publishing Group; 2000:55-61.

11. Shields MB. *Textbook of Glaucoma*. 4th ed. Baltimore, Md: Williams and Wilkins; 1998:46-71.

12. Grant WM, Schuman JS. Tonometry and tonography. In: Epstein DL, Allingham RR, Schuman JS, eds. *Chandler and Grant's Glaucoma*. 4th ed. Baltimore, Md: Williams and Wilkins; 1997:41-50.

13. American Academy of Ophthalmology. *Glaucoma. Basic and Clinical Science Course 2003-2004*. San Francisco, Calif: American Academy of Ophthalmology; 2003:14-48.

14. Brandt JD, Beiser JA, Kass MA, Gordon MO. Central corneal thickness in the Ocular Hypertension Treatment Study (OHTS). *Ophthalmology*. 2001;108:1779-1788.

15. Herndon L. Rethinking pachymetry and intraocular pressure. *Rev Ophthalmol*. 2002;July:88-90.

16. Ehlers N, Bramsen T, Sperling S. Applanation tonometry and central corneal thickness. *Acta Ophthalmol (Copenh)*. 1975;53:34-43.

17. Shimmyo M, Ross AJ, Moy A, Mostafavi R. Intraocular pressure, Goldmann applanation tension, corneal thickness, and corneal curvature in Caucasians, Asians, Hispanics, and African Americans. *Am J Ophthalmol*. 2003;136:603-613.

18. Herndon LW, Weizer JS, Stinnett SS. Central corneal thickness as a risk factor for advanced glaucoma damage. *Arch Ophthalmol*. 2004;122:17-21.

19. Epstein DL. Examination of the eye. In: Epstein DL, Allingham RR, Schuman JS, eds. *Chandler and Grant's Glaucoma*. 4th ed. Baltimore, Md: Williams and Wilkins; 1997:33-40.

20. Foster PJ, Johnson GJ. Primary angle closure: classification and clinical features. In: Hitchings RA, ed. *Glaucoma*. London: BMJ Publishing Group; 2000:145-152.

21. Forbes M. Gonioscopy with corneal indentation. A method for distinguishing between appositional closure and synechial closure. *Arch Ophthalmol*. 1966;76:488-492.

22. Shields MB. *Textbook of Glaucoma*. 4th ed. Baltimore, Md: Williams and Wilkins; 1998:72-107.

23. Jonas J, Garaway-Heath T. Primary glaucomas: optic disc features. In: Hitchings RA, ed. *Glaucoma*. London: BMJ Publishing Group; 2000:29-38.

24. Drance SM. Disc hemorrhages in the glaucomas. *Surv Ophthalmol*. 1989;33:331-337.

25. Greenfield DS, Siatkowski RM, Glaser JS, Schatz NJ, Parrish RK 2nd. The cupped disc. Who needs neuroimaging? *Ophthalmology*. 1998;105:1866-1874.

26. Leske MC, Heijl A, Hussein M, Bengtsson B, Hyman L, Komaroff E. Factors for glaucoma progression and the effect of treatment: the Early Manifest Glaucoma Trial. *Arch Ophthalmol*. 2003;121:48-56.

27. Sommer A, Katz J, Quigley HA, et al. Clinically detectable nerve fiber atrophy precedes the onset of glaucomatous field loss. *Arch Ophthalmol*. 1991;109:77-83.

28. Epstein DL. Examination of the optic nerve. In: Epstein DL, Allingham RR, Schuman JS, eds. *Chandler and Grant's Glaucoma*. 4th ed. Baltimore, Md: Williams and Wilkins; 1997:84-103.

2

3

Visual Field and Ancillary Testing

Perimetry

Pathologic cupping and optic nerve atrophy produce visible changes on optic disc examination that correspond to specific visual field defects.[1] As noted, these changes may precede detectable field loss. The type of pathologic cupping and its associated disc changes should correspond to the type and location of the visual field loss. For example, when the disc atrophy and pathologic cupping are located inferiorly and temporally, the corresponding glaucomatous field defect should present as an upper nasal step defect, a superior arcuate/Bjerrum scotoma, or a combination of both. If the enlargement of the cup is situated superiorly, the corresponding field defect would be an inferior arcuate/Bjerrum scotoma, an inferior nasal step, or both.[1] Moreover, defects in the retinal nerve fiber layer (RNFL) may, in fact, provide the earliest reliable evidence of field loss in glaucoma.[2]

Neuroretinal rim thinning and/or defects in the RNFL correspond well with detectable visual field loss. Thus optic disc, RNFL, and visual field examinations are essential components in the management of glaucoma. These discernible changes may have their greatest value in the diagnosis and management of early-stage glaucoma. As noted in the following section, a variety of techniques have been developed to test for visual field defects under photopic conditions.

Static Threshold Testing

Threshold testing involves the differential light sensitivity at which a stimulus of a given size and duration of presentation is seen approximately 50% of the time (ie, the dimmest spot detected during testing).[3] Static testing employs a stationary object presented at different locations with the intensity increased or decreased in a systematic manner to establish the threshold value. The light intensity is gradually increased from a subthreshold level to an intensity level that is discernible to the patient. The test may be performed manually, but it is usually obtained by an automated machine. The test results can be represented symbolically, graphically, or numerically.[4]

The most common threshold test program in static perimetry measures about 54 to 76 points on the retina in the central 24° to 30° of the field with a 6° grid between test locations. The 6° grid can, however, miss small glaucomatous defects as well as the blind spot. Commonly used programs for measuring the central 24° to 30° are the Octopus 32 and Humphrey 24-2 and 30-2.[2,3] The Humphrey 30-2 threshold test pattern is shown in **Figure 3**.**1**. If visual field loss close to central fixation is known or anticipated, specific programs that measure the central 10° (eg, Humphrey 10-2) should be selected. In addition, a number of other advanced perimetry techniques (described below) hold the promise of detecting visual field defects more reliably and at an earlier stage.

- **Swedish Interactive Threshold Algorithm (SITA)**

The Swedish Interactive Threshold Algorithm is an improved software program for performing full-threshold automated perimetry. The stimulus source is the same as for standard perimetry, but uses an intelli-

FIGURE 3.1 — CENTRAL 30-2 THRESHOLD TEST PATTERN: RIGHT EYE

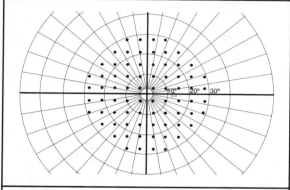

The Field Analyzer Primer. San Leandro, Calif: Allergan Humphrey; 1989.

gent algorithm to continuously estimate threshold values and errors.[5,6] SITA also incorporates a variety of information that includes patient age, normative data, knowledge of abnormal test patterns, and patient responses over the test interval. The SITA program provides the same accuracy as standard methods, but it reduces the testing time by approximately 50% with less variability in threshold values.[6]

■ Short-Wavelength Automated Perimetry (SWAP)

There are three main types of retinal ganglion cells (RGCs) that differ in their response to light stimuli:

- Parvocellular cells that respond to high spatial resolution
- Magnocellular cells that respond to low spatial frequency
- Bistratified ganglion cells, which are stimulated by blue light and suppressed by yellow light.[6]

The SWAP algorithm utilizes a blue light stimulus and a yellow background to activate the bistratified ganglion cells while bleaching out the red and green cones. This technique may predict glaucomatous field loss 2 to 5 years earlier than standard perimetry.[6,7] SWAP can also detect larger defects, but it requires significantly more testing time than standard perimetry and the bright light is disturbing to many patients. The technique also has a higher threshold variability than that of standard perimetry.[8]

■ Interpretation of Visual Fields

The complexity of data derived from visual field testing by various perimetry methods requires careful interpretation based on a number of parameters, which are outlined in **Table 3.1**. Computerized statistic programs available with many perimeters are quite valuable for analyzing the data.

Kinetic Testing

Kinetic perimetry involves moving a target (light stimulus) from a nonseeing area toward a seeing area. The location at which the patient first visualizes the target is recorded. The procedure is usually performed manually and determines the boundaries of the visual field at a given threshold, from which an isopter can be drawn.[2-4]

■ Goldmann Perimetry

The original standard for perimetry is the Goldmann perimeter. It consists of a uniformly illuminated bowl and evaluates central and peripheral visual fields with targets of varying size and intensity.[4] With the Goldmann perimeter, a selective screening technique tests only those areas with the highest probability of glaucomatous defects. The central visual field is tested by suprathreshold static procedures, and the peripheral field is tested with kinetic perimetry. These techniques have been shown to have a high degree of sensitivity and specificity.[2]

■ Tangent Screen

The tangent screen is a flat black panel with a central fixation point on which the central 30° of the visual field can be evaluated. Both static and kinetic techniques can be used to test the central field. The main advantage is its ability to detect the relative size and location of visual field defects. However, tangent screen testing is manual and qualitative rather than quantitative, and it does not provide good reproducibility for monitoring changes and progression in patients with glaucoma.[2,4]

■ Frequency-Doubling Technology (FDT)

FDT perimetry relies on a frequency-doubling illusion that activates retinal magnocellular ganglion cells. In this test, the patient sees varying shades of gray patterns alternating at high frequencies, and responds to seeing a pattern of bars.[6,8] Defects in the magnocellular ganglion cells are thought to occur early in glaucoma, and FDT may provide early diagnosis of the disease. FDT compares well with standard perimetry in detecting glaucomatous damage and provides abnormal results in glaucoma suspects. It is faster than standard perimetry and appears to have high patient acceptance. At present, FDT appears to be more valuable as a screening test rather than as a method for longitudinal visual field evaluations.[6]

■ Confrontational Visual Field Testing

Confrontational visual field testing may be used to quickly detect gross defects in the visual field. This technique has particular value in patients with dense ocular media such as cataracts and in patients unable to respond to other methods of perimetry. Also, it may

TABLE 3.1 — PARAMETERS IN INTERPRETATION OF AUTOMATED STATIC PERIMETRY	
Parameter	**Significance**
Visual field indices	Statistical analysis of threshold data: • Mean sensitivity (an average of all threshold values) • Mean deviation (averages of all the differences between each threshold value and the age-corrected normal) • Pattern Standard Deviation (standard deviation of all the differences between each threshold value and the age-corrected normal) • Corrected Pattern Standard Deviation (pattern standard deviation adjusted for short-term fluctuation)
Reliability indices	• Fixation losses (should be <20%) • False positives (should be <33%) • False negatives (intratest failure to respond to stimulus >9 dB from previously determined threshold; should be <33%)
Threshold variability	• Short-term fluctuation (intratest standard deviation of differences between repeated threshold values at 10 preselected points; should be <2.5 dB) • Long-term fluctuation (physiological variation in visual status; usually generalized rather than focal [differentiate from progression of disease])

Glaucoma hemifield test	• Calculates differences of thresholds of mirror-image preselected groups of points in upper and lower hemifields for comparison with normal database. Determines whether differences are abnormal, borderline or normal
Single-field evaluation	• Quality (assess reliability indices) • Assess probabilities of mean deviation (MD), pattern standard deviation, corrected pattern standard deviation (CPSD), and glaucoma hemifield test (GHT) • Assess greyscale pattern of defect(s) • Normal photopic thresholds decrease from center to periphery • Cluster of ≥2 points depressed ≥5 dB compared with surrounding points is suspicious • Artifacts—lens rim, incorrect lens power, cloverleaf pattern (inattention) false-positive and/or false-negative >33% (unreliable although high false-negative occurs in glaucoma)
Series of fields	• Assess changes in mean deviation and pattern standard deviation • New scotoma (reproducible depression of a previously normal point ≥11 dB or 2 adjacent points by ≥5 dB • Enlargement of existing scotoma (reproducible depression of an adjacent point ≥ 9 dB) • Deepening of existing scotoma (reproducible depression of a point in an existing scotoma ≥7 dB)

Adapted from: Shields MB. *Textbook of Glaucoma*. 4th ed. Baltimore, Md: Williams and Wilkins; 1998:108–136; and American Academy of Ophthalmology. *Glaucoma. Basic and Clinical Science Course 2003-2004*. San Francisco, Calif: American Academy of Ophthalmology; 2003:48–71.

be used to assess the location and to estimate the size of a small residual field in a patient with late-stage glaucoma.[4]

Glaucomatous Visual Field Defects

Visual field defects bear names that relate to their appearance on plots of kinetic visual field charts.

■ Arcuate Scotoma

This defect occurs in the arcuate or Bjerrum area that corresponds to the arcuate retinal nerve fibers (**Figure 3.2**).[2] Visual loss in this area commonly occurs in glaucoma and is associated with a tendency for early development of glaucomatous damage in the inferior and superior temporal poles of the optic nerve head (ONH).[9,10]

■ Paracentral Scotomas

Paracentral scotomas develop within the arcuate area and are discrete or localized losses in retinal response. They begin as intermittent, shallow depressions, but as glaucomatous damage progresses, paracentral scotomas enlarge and ultimately become arcuate scotomas.[4,11]

■ Nasal Step

The rate of retinal nerve fiber deterioration is usually different in the upper and lower segments of the eye. Therefore, a distinct steplike defect manifests as either discontinuity or depression along an isopter above or below the horizontal nasal raphe.[2-4]

■ Temporal Wedge/Step

A wedge-shaped defect may extend temporally from the blind spot. The defect likely represents damage to the RNFL bundle(s) in the superonasal and/or inferonasal nerve region.[3]

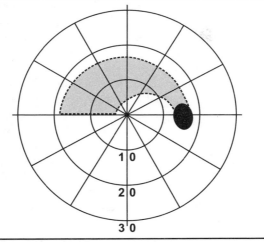

FIGURE 3.2 — ARCUATE OR BJERRUM VISUAL FIELD AREA

1 0

2 0

3 0

The arcuate or Bjerrum area is defined by the dotted lines.

Adapted from: Shields MB. *Textbook of Glaucoma*. 4th ed. Baltimore, Md: Williams and Wilkins; 1998:114.

■ Altitudinal Defect

This dense horizontal defect results from enlargement of a superior or inferior arcuate scotoma by extension inward to the horizontal midline and outward to the peripheral boundary of the visual field. If severe, the defect may extend close to or even split fixation.

Retinal Nerve Fiber Layer Thickness

A reduction in the thickness of the RNFL by as little as 10 to 20 microns is a strong predictor of visual field loss.[12] Therefore, it is important to be able to detect and objectively quantify changes in RNFL thickness. One method for achieving this is optical coherence tomography (OCT). This technique achieves high-resolution cross-sectional imaging of the RNFL with low coherence light, and it is a highly accurate method of determining thickness measurements for both normal and glaucomatous eyes.[13] OCT is similar to B-mode ultrasound, but because it uses light instead of sound, there is no need for direct contact with the eye. Moreover, the technique provides imaging of both anterior and posterior segments.[12]

Scanning laser ophthalmoscopy is also used to determine RNFL thickness. One such technique is scanning laser polarimetry using the Nerve Fiber Analyser—NFA or GDx, from Laser Diagnostic Technologies, Inc.[14] This device uses a polarized, near-infrared laser beam to scan the fundus at the ONH and peripapillary retina. The change in polarization of the beam reflected from the RNFL is correlated with the thickness of the layer. Measurements have been shown to be valid and reproducible.[14]

Optic Disc Topography

Confocal scanning laser ophthalmoscopy using the Heidelberg Retina Tomograph (HRT, Heidleberg Engineering) provides objective topographic measurements of the ONH.[14] The HRT utilizes confocal imaging and focuses a laser beam in a given plane at the fundus. The device limits imaging only to the plane in focus and produces a series of optical sections at various axial depths. In this manner, a topographic map of the optic disc, optic cup, and neuroretinal rim can be obtained and analyzed for serial glaucomatous changes.[14]

■ Optic Nerve Head Blood Flow

Scanning laser Doppler flowmetry allows for the noninvasive assessment of ocular hemodynamics in the ONH of patients with open-angle glaucoma (OAG). The technology permits direct quantitative measurements of blood flow in the ONH and peripapillary regions in a valid and reproducible manner.[15]

Visual Function

- **Color Vision**

A decline in color sensitivity may occur before visual field loss in glaucoma. This loss in color sensitivity occurs mainly in the blue-sensitive pathways. These pathways are minimally involved in the sensation of brightness or visual acuity, which may account for the fact that standard tests often fail to detect a diminution in color vision.[2] Color abnormalities in early glaucoma appear to be related to RNFL loss. The technique of SWAP (discussed earlier) can detect color vision loss associated with glaucoma since it uses a blue target on a yellow background. Early GON may be correlated with deficits uncovered by the SWAP technique prior to detection by standard perimetry.[2]

- **Multifocal Visually Evoked Potentials**

Visually evoked potentials (VEPs) have been found to be abnormal in glaucoma, and a reduced response to high-frequency flicker VEPs corresponds to the degree of glaucomatous deterioration.[2] The multifocal VEP may detect abnormalities in visual function in patients with early to mild glaucomatous damage and normal results on static achromatic automated perimetry. However, the reverse is true as well.[16]

- **Contrast Sensitivity**

Early central and peripheral visual field losses can be detected by measuring the degree of contrast necessary to distinguish between adjacent visual stimuli in glaucoma patients. These losses may be detected before those found with standard perimetry.[2] Spatial contrast sensitivity relies on sine wave gratings that require patients to detect striped patterns at different degrees of contrast and spatial frequencies. In temporal contrast sensitivity, the patient is required to perceive visual stimuli at different degrees of contrast and flicker frequencies.

- ■ **Amsler Grid**

In patients with visual field loss close to central fixation (ie, split fixation), Amsler grid testing may be useful in monitoring for potential progression.

Blood Flow Testing

The normal eye compensates for a decrease in perfusion pressure as a result of elevated intraocular pressure (IOP), as seen with laser Doppler blood flow measurements of the ONH.[17] These same measurement techniques show reduced flow velocity in glaucomatous eyes.[18,19] However, patients with OAG may show significant improvement in ONH blood flow in response to aggressive lowering of IOP of >20% from baseline levels (as measured by scanning laser Doppler flowmetry).[20] Interestingly, patients with OH did not demonstrate this response.

Genetic Testing

Family history is an important risk factor for the development of primary open-angle glaucoma (POAG). The Baltimore Eye Survey reported a 3.7 times greater risk of having POAG when a sibling also had the disease; the risk was 2.2 times greater when a parent had the disease.[21] It is now possible to perform glaucoma screening in families for the presence of a causative gene mutation.[22] This screening requires identification of three affected family members from at least two generations. The studies involve candidate gene and random genome search techniques and require careful family phenotyping and history taking for glaucoma. A number of genetic loci for various forms of glaucoma have been discovered. These include juvenile OAG, adult-onset POAG, normal-tension glaucoma, and the congenital glaucomas.[23,24]

REFERENCES

1. Epstein DL. Examination of the optic nerve. In: Epstein DL, Allingham RR, Schuman JS, eds. *Chandler and Grant's Glaucoma*. 4th ed. Baltimore, Md: Williams and Wilkins; 1997:84-103.

2. Shields MB. *Textbook of Glaucoma*. 4th ed. Baltimore, Md: Williams and Wilkins; 1998:108-136.

3. American Academy of Ophthalmology. *Glaucoma. Basic and Clinical Science Course 2003-2004*. San Francisco, Calif: American Academy of Ophthalmology; 2003:48-71.

4. Allingham RR. Visual fields and their relationship to the optic nerve. In: Epstein DL, Allingham RR, Schuman JS, eds. *Chandler and Grant's Glaucoma*. 4th ed. Baltimore, Md: Williams and Wilkins; 1997:120-128.

5. Johnson CA. Recent developments in automated perimetry in glaucoma diagnosis and management. *Curr Opin Ophthalmol*. 2002;13:77-84.

6. Delgado MF, Nguyen NT, Cox TA, et al. Automated perimetry: a report by the American Academy of Ophthalmology. *Ophthalmology*. 2002;109:2362-2374.

7. Girkin CA, Emdadi A, Sample PA, et al. Short-wavelength automated perimetry and standard perimetry in the detection of progressive optic disc cupping. *Arch Ophthalmol*. 2000;118:1231-1236.

8. Heijl A. Glaucoma perimetry. In: Hitchings RA, ed. *Glaucoma*. London: BMJ Publishing Group; 2000:39-54.

9. Gramer E, Gerlach R, Krieglstein GK, Leydhecker W. Topography of early glaucomatous visual defects in computerized perimetry. *Klin Monatsbl Augenheikld*. 1982;180:515-523.

10. Harrington DO. The Bjerrum scotomas. *Am J Ophthalmol*. 1965;59:646.

11. Mikelberg FS, Drance SM. The mode of progression of visual defects in glaucoma. *Am J Ophthalmol.* 1984;98:443-445.

12. Shuman JS. Imaging of the optic nerve head and nerve fiber layer in glaucoma. In: Epstein DL, Allingham RR, Schuman JS, eds. *Chandler and Grant's Glaucoma.* 4th ed. Baltimore, Md: Williams and Wilkins; 1997:104-119.

13. Blumenthal EZ, Williams JM, Weinreb RN, Girkin CA, Berry CC, Zangwill LM. Reproducibility of nerve fiber layer thickness measurements by use of optical coherence tomography. *Ophthalmology.* 2000;107:2278-2282.

14. Garway-Heath T. The identification of progression in cupping of the optic disc. In: Hitchings RA, ed. *Glaucoma.* London: BMJ Publishing Group; 2000:128-138.

15. Michelson G, Schmauss B, Langhans MJ, Harazny J, Groh MJ. Principle, validity, and reliability of scanning laser Doppler flowmetry. *J Glaucoma.* 1996;5:99-105.

16. Hood DC, Thienprasiddhi P, Greenstein VC, et al. Detecting early to mild glaucomatous damage: a comparison of the multifocal VEP and automated perimetry. *Invest Ophthalmol Vis Sci.* 2004;45:492-498.

17. Riva CE, Grunwald JE, Sinclair SH. Laser Doppler measurement of relative blood velocity in the human optic nerve head. *Invest Ophthalmol Vis Sci.* 1982;22:241-248.

18. Costa VP, Sergott RC, Smith M, et al. Color Doppler imaging in glaucoma patients with asymmetric optic cups. *J Glaucoma.* 1994;3:S91.

19. Rojanapongpun P, Drance SM, Morrison BJ. Ophthalmic artery flow velocity in glaucomatous and normal subjects. *Br J Ophthalmol.* 1993;77:25-29.

20. Hafez AS, Bizzarro RL, Rivard M, Lesk MR. Changes in optic nerve head blood flow after therapeutic intraocular pressure reduction in glaucoma patients and ocular hypertensives. *Ophthalmology.* 2003;110:201-210.

21. Tielsch JM, Katz J, Sommer A, Quigley HA, Javitt JC. Family history and risk of primary open angle glaucoma. The Baltimore Eye Survey. *Arch Ophthalmol.* 1994;112:69-73.

22. Sarfarazi M. Recent advances in molecular genetics of glaucomas. *Hum Mol Genet.* 1997;6:1667-1677.

23. Child AH. Genetic screening for glaucoma. In: Hitchings RA, ed. *Glaucoma.* London: BMJ Publishing Group; 2000:22-28.

24. WuDunn D. Genetic basis of glaucoma. *Curr Opin Ophthalmol.* 2002;13:55-60.

3

TABLE 4.1 — SUMMARY OF INCIDENCE AND PREVALENCE DATA FOR OPEN-ANGLE GLAUCOMA		
Study	Incidence for All Ages	Prevalence
Quigley[1]	1.1 per 100,000/y among whites 3.9 per 100,000/y among blacks	1.55% among whites over 40* 4.6% among blacks over 40†
Baltimore Eye Survey[2]	Not applicable	1.29% among whites over 40 4.3% among blacks over 40
The Beaver Dam Eye Study[3]	Not applicable	2.9% among whites

* Median age-adjusted prevalence.
† Overall age-adjusted prevalence.

1. Quigley HA, Vitale S. Models of open-angle glaucoma prevalence and incidence in the United States. *Invest Ophthalmol Vis Sci.* 1997;38:83-91.
2. Tielsch JM, Sommer A, Katz J, et al. Racial variations in the prevalence of primary open-angle glaucoma. The Baltimore Eye Survey. *JAMA.*1991;266:369-374.
3. Klein BEK, Klein R, Sponsel WE, et al. Prevalence of glaucoma. The Beaver Dam Eye Study. *Ophthalmology.* 1992;99:1499-1504.

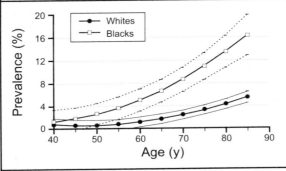

FIGURE 4.1 — ESTIMATED PREVALENCE OF OPEN-ANGLE GLAUCOMA AMONG BOTH BLACK AND WHITE PERSONS BY AGE

The 95% confidence limits are indicated by flanking lines. The model estimated in white persons that the relationship was best approximated by prevalence = (1.59×10^{-2}) − $(1.14 \times 10^{-3}) \times$ (age − 30) + $(3.39 \times 10^{-5}) \times$ (age − 30)^2. In black persons, it estimated that the relationship was best approximated by prevalence = (1.18×10^{-2}) + $(3.94 \times 10^{-4}) \times$ (age − 30) + $(5.73 \times 10^{-5}) \times$ (age − 30)^2. Where the model predicted values of prevalence that were < zero, we used zero for the prevalence.

Quigley HA, Vitale S. *Invest Ophthalmol Vis Sci.* 1997;38:83-91.

field, cup/disc ratio, and IOP. Of note was the finding that the frequency of combinations of abnormal risk factors for defining glaucoma increased with every decade. The prevalence of OAG was 2.9%, a figure somewhat higher than for the white population in the Baltimore Eye Survey. An especially important finding was that approximately one third of patients diagnosed with OAG presented with normal levels of IOP (ie, normal-pressure glaucoma [NPG]).

The Rotterdam Study assessed the prevalence of POAG in a single-center, prospective, population-based cohort study.[6] Over 3000 participants were ex-

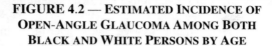

FIGURE 4.2 — ESTIMATED INCIDENCE OF OPEN-ANGLE GLAUCOMA AMONG BOTH BLACK AND WHITE PERSONS BY AGE

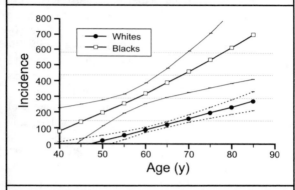

Estimated incidence of open-angle glaucoma for both black and white persons by age (per 100,000 persons/year). The 95% confidence limits are indicated by flanking lines.

Quigley HA, Vitale S. *Invest Ophthalmol Vis Sci.* 1997;38:83-91.

amined according to standard protocols, including perimetry. While the overall prevalence of POAG was 1.1%, the age-specific prevalence figures increased from 0.2% in the 55- to 59-year age group to 3.3% in the 85- to 89-year age group. Of the patients not diagnosed previously with POAG, 38.9% had IOPs ≤21 mm Hg (ie, NPG).

The Barbados Eye Study measured the 4-year risk of OAG in a random sample of over 3000 black residents in the West Indies.[7] The 4-year risk of OAG was 2.2%; incidence rates during that 4-year period increased from 1.2% at ages 40 to 49 to 4.2% at ages 70 and older. Although IOP increased the risk of developing glaucoma, approximately 50% of newly diagnosed cases of OAG had baseline pressures ≤21 mm Hg (ie, NPG). The results confirmed again the high risk of OAG in populations of African origin, especially in older age groups.

The Blue Mountains Eye Study determined the prevalence of OAG and ocular hypertension (OH) in approximately 3600 residents (≥49 years of age) in an Australian community.[8] The overall prevalence of OAG was 3.0%, with one half of the cases newly diagnosed. An exponential rise in the prevalence rates was observed with increasing age. In addition, OH was present in another 3.7% of the population.

Finally, Proyecto VER assessed the prevalence of glaucoma in a population-based sample of Hispanic adults 40 years or older in Arizona.[9] The age-specific prevalence of OAG increased exponentially from 0.5% at 41 to 49 years of age to 12.63% in those ≥80 years of age. Only 38% of the persons identified with OAG knew of their diagnosis before the study. In addition, OAG was the leading cause of bilateral blindness.

In conclusion, the above population-based studies have strongly implicated age as a major risk factor for the development of POAG. The increased prevalence of the disease among patients of African and Hispanic heritage is clearly noted. With increasing levels of IOP, the risk of developing OAG also increases dramatically. However, a significant number of patients diagnosed with OAG (ie, 25% to 40%) present with normal levels of IOP.

REFERENCES

1. Quigley HA. Number of people with glaucoma worldwide. *Br J Ophthalmol.* 1996;80:389-393.

2. Quigley HA, Vitale S. Models of open-angle glaucoma prevalence and incidence in the United States. *Invest Ophthalmol Vis Sci.* 1997;38:83-91.

3. Tielsch JM, Sommer A, Katz J, Royall RM, Quigley HA, Javitt J. Racial variations in the prevalence of primary open-angle glaucoma. The Baltimore Eye Survey. *JAMA.* 1991;266:369-374.

4. Sommer A, Tielsch JM, Katz J, et al. Relationship between intraocular pressure and primary open angle glaucoma among white and black Americans. The Baltimore Eye Survey. *Arch Ophthalmol.* 1991;109:1090-1095.

5. Klein BE, Klein R, Sponsel WE, et al. Prevalence of glaucoma. The Beaver Dam Eye Study. *Ophthalmology.* 1992;99:1499-1504.

6. Dielemans I, Vingerling JR, Wolfs RC, Hofman A, Grobbee DE, de Jong PT. The prevalence of primary open-angle glaucoma in a population-based study in The Netherlands. The Rotterdam Study. *Ophthalmology.* 1994;101:1851-1855.

7. Leske MC, Connell AM, Wu SY, et al. Incidence of open-angle glaucoma: the Barbados Eye Studies. The Barbados Eye Studies Group. *Arch Ophthalmol.* 2001;119:89-95.

8. Mitchell P, Smith W, Attebo K, Healey PR. Prevalence of open-angle glaucoma in Australia. The Blue Mountains Eye Study. *Ophthalmology.* 1996;103:1661-1669.

9. Quigley HA, West SK, Rodriquez J, Munoz B, Klein R, Snyder R. The prevalence of glaucoma in a population-based study of Hispanic subjects: Proyecto VER. *Arch Ophthalmol.* 2001;119:1819-1826.

5

Etiology: Primary
Open-Angle Glaucoma

Intraocular Pressure—Aqueous Humor Outflow Obstruction

Conventional aqueous humor outflow occurs via a drainage system that includes the trabecular meshwork (uveal meshwork, corneoscleral meshwork, and juxtacanalicular tissue), Schlemm's canal, intrascleral aqueous veins (or collector channels), and episcleral veins. The aqueous eventually drains into the anterior ciliary and superior ophthalmic veins.[1] This conventional outflow pathway accounts for 83% to 96% of total aqueous outflow and is dependent on intraocular pressure (IOP).[2,3] The remaining aqueous outflow occurs via the uveoscleral, or nonconventional, pathway and is believed to be independent of IOP.[1,2,4] However, recent studies suggest that uveoscleral outflow may account for as much as 40% to 50% of aqueous humor outflow in normal eyes.[5]

The difference between the IOP and episcleral venous pressure values is attributed to normal resistance to aqueous humor outflow. It is commonly accepted that the major portion of normal resistance resides in the trabecular meshwork–Schlemm's canal complex.[6,7] Increased resistance in the trabecular meshwork and Schlemm's canal is usually expressed as a reciprocal decrease in aqueous humor outflow facility that causes increased IOP. Several mechanisms have been proposed for this increase in resistance[7-9]:

- Obstruction of the trabecular network by foreign matter
- Loss of trabecular endothelial cells

- Decrease in permeability of the trabecular meshwork
- Loss of normal phagocytic activity (acts as a self-cleaning mechanism)
- Increased resistance of the inner wall of Schlemm's canal and partial collapse of the canal.

Optic Neuropathy

Although the etiology of glaucomatous optic neuropathy (GON) is multifactorial, elevated IOP is a major risk factor for its development. Ischemia in the optic nerve head has been shown to contribute to the pathogenesis of GON,[10] and blood flow is known to be affected by IOP. In addition, blood flow is dependent on ocular perfusion pressure, which is equal to mean arterial blood pressure minus IOP. Thus elevated IOP will result in diminished perfusion pressure and decreased blood flow in susceptible eyes (wherein autoregulation has been compromised). Defects in the normal autoregulation process—which maintains a constant blood flow in response to changes in perfusion pressure—have been associated with GON.[10]

Elevated IOP also causes structural and functional changes in the lamina cribrosa, through which the optic nerve axons pass (**Figure 5.1**).[11] For example, elevated IOP results in contortion of the lamina cribrosa, thereby leading to compression of the axon bundles passing through the lamina and subsequent nerve damage. This structural change also diminishes retrograde axoplasmic transport of nerve growth factors, thereby further contributing to atrophy of the axons. Ultimately, there is a corresponding secondary reduction in blood supply to the atrophied nerve fibers.[7]

IOP-independent apoptosis, or programmed cell death, is a significant cause of retinal ganglion cell (RGC) loss in GON.[12] This biologic process may be the final pathway in RGC death regardless of the ini-

FIGURE 5.1 — OPTIC NERVE HEAD REGIONS

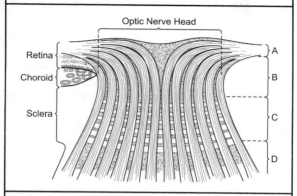

A) Surface nerve fiber layer; B) prelaminar region;
C) lamina cribrosa region; D) retrolaminar region.

Adapted from: Shields MB. *Textbook of Glaucoma*. 4th ed. Baltimore, Md: Williams and Wilkins; 1998:73.

tiating insult. Although elevated IOP is one of the main initiating factors, apoptosis may occur independently of elevated IOP (as a result of other stimuli such as ischemia, traumatic injury, and genetic influences). For example, an insult to the optic nerve may cause the release of toxic substances that initiate apoptosis via activation of apoptosis-induction genes. These genes are present in every RGC, but are normally inactivated by various prosurvival factors. In the presence of toxic insults to the RGCs that upset this aspect of normal cellular homeostasis, the process of apoptosis may be initiated.

Genetic Factors

A genetic causal factor in glaucoma has been theorized based on studies showing an increased incidence of primary open-angle glaucoma (POAG) in relatives of patients with known glaucoma, and the occurrence of familial POAG.[12] GLC1 is the code assigned to the causal genes that have been discovered for POAG. Mutations in the myocilin (MYOC) gene has been demonstrated to account for up to 4% of known cases of POAG, as well as a much higher percentage of cases of juvenile open-angle glaucoma.[13] A number of other genetic loci for POAG have also been reported.[14]

Optineurin, or optic neuropathy–inducing protein, was recently identified as a causative gene for autosomal dominantly inherited adult-onset POAG.[15] Sequence alterations in optineurin were found in 16.7% of families with hereditary POAG; the majority of the patients had normal levels of IOP. Optineurin, present in the trabecular meshwork, was found to be significantly upregulated after 2, 4, and 7 days of sustained elevated IOP. Its expression also appears to be increased 2.3 times by tumor necrosis factor-alpha (TNF-α) and 2.6 times by prolonged dexamethasone treatment.[15,16] Finally, a number of other heritable genetic disorders with associated glaucoma, such as aniridia and Axenfeld-Rieger syndrome, have been characterized.[14]

Systemic Factors

Vasospastic conditions that may cause secondary ischemia have been suggested as factors in the etiology of GON. Migraine, which is associated with temporary alterations in blood flow and peripheral vasospasm, may be a risk factor for normal-tension glaucoma (NTG).[17,18] It has been theorized that vasospasm leads to focal regions of ischemia that compromise optic nerve head perfusion. However, a causal association has not been clearly delineated. Another vasospastic condition with a potential link to glaucoma is Raynaud's phenomenon. An association has been described between the frequent occurrence of cold hands and the visual field loss found in optic neuropathy; the corresponding optic nerve excavation resembled that of NTG.[19,20]

REFERENCES

1. Krupin T. *Manual of Glaucoma: Diagnosis and Management.* New York, NY: Churchill Livingston; 1988:1-5.

2. Bill A, Phillips CI. Uveoscleral drainage of aqueous humour in human eyes. *Exp Eye Res.* 1971;12:275-281.

3. Joscon VL, Sears ML. Experimental aqueous perfusion in enucleated human eyes. Results after obstruction of Schlemm's canal. *Arch Ophthalmol.* 1971;86:65-71.

4. Bill A. The drainage of aqueous humor via Schlemm's canal and uveoscleral routes. *Ophthal Res.* 1980;12:130.

5. Toris CB, Yablonski ME, Wang YL, Camras CB. Aqueous humor dynamics in the aging human eye. *Am J Ophthalmol.* 1999;127:407-412.

6. Shields MB. *Textbook of Glaucoma.* 4th ed. Baltimore, Md: Williams and Wilkins; 1998:1-31.

7. Hoskins HD Jr, Kass MA. *Becker-Shaffer's Diagnosis and Therapy of the Glaucomas.* 6th ed. St. Louis, Mo: CV Mosby Co; 1989:49.

8. Scheie HG, Fleischauer HW. Idiopathic atrophy of the epithelial layers of the iris and ciliary body. *Arch Ophthalmol.* 1958;59:565.

9. Quigley HA, Addicks EM. Scanning electron microscopy of trabeculectomy specimens from eyes with open-angle glaucoma. *Am J Ophthalmol.* 1980;90:854-857.

10. Hayreh SS. Factors influencing blood flow in the optic nerve head. *J Glaucoma.* 1997;6:412-425.

11. Emery JM, Landis D, Paton D, Boniuk M, Craig JM. The lamina cribrosa on normal and glaucomatous human eyes. *Trans Am Acad Ophthalmol Otolaryngol.* 1974;78:290-297.

12. Sherwood MS, Brandt JD. Future scientific directions. In: American Academy of Ophthalmology, ed. *A LEO Clinical Update Course on Glaucoma*. San Francisco, Calif: American Academy of Ophthalmology; 2000.

13. Fingert JH, Stone EM, Sheffield VC, Alward WL. Myocilin glaucoma. *Surv Ophthalmol*. 2002;47:547-561.

14. WuDunn D. Genetic basis of glaucoma. *Curr Opin Ophthalmol*. 2002;13:55-60.

15. Rezaie T, Child A, Hitchings R, et al. Adult-onset primary open-angle glaucoma caused by mutations in optineurin. *Science*. 2002;295:1077-1079.

16. Vittitow J, Borras T. Expression of optineurin, a glaucoma-linked gene, is influenced by elevated intraocular pressure. *Biochem Biophys Res Commun*. 2002;298:67-74.

17. Corbett JJ, Phelps CD, Eslinger P, Montague PR. The neurologic evaluation of patients with low-tension glaucoma. *Invest Ophthalmol Vis Sci*. 1985;26:1101-1104.

18. Phelps CD, Corbett JJ. Migraine and low-tension glaucoma. A case-control study. *Invest Ophthalmol Vis Sci*. 1985;26:1105.

19. Gasser P, Flammer J. Influence of vasospasm on visual function. *Doc Ophthalmol*. 1987;66:3-18.

20. Gasser P, Flammer J. Blood-cell velocity in the nailfold capillaries of patients with normal-tension and high-tension glaucoma. *Am J Ophthalmol*. 1991;111:585-588.

6

Natural History: Primary Open-Angle Glaucoma

Ocular Hypertension Conversion to Primary Open-Angle Glaucoma

Although glaucoma is a multifactorial disease, it is widely recognized that elevated intraocular pressure (IOP) is a major risk factor for the development of glaucomatous optic neuropathy (GON). Current estimates suggest that 3 to 6 million people in the United States have elevated IOP without detectable signs of glaucoma on routine ophthalmic examination.[1] Epidemiologic data (Chapter 4, *Epidemiology: Primary Open-Angle Glaucoma*) indicate that approximately 10% of the 66.8 million people with glaucoma worldwide will experience bilateral blindness.

In the Ocular Hypertension Treatment Study (OHTS), 1636 patients with ocular hypertension but no signs of GON were randomized to IOP-lowering therapy or observation.[2] After 60 months, the cumulative probability of developing primary open-angle glaucoma (POAG) was more than twice as high for the control group compared with the treatment group (9.4% vs 4.4%, respectively). Thus the OHTS results indicate a need for earlier treatment in patients with elevated IOP with moderate or severe risk of developing glaucoma. This may be especially pertinent since GON often precedes detectable visual field loss in these patients.[3]

Early Manifest Open-Angle Glaucoma

The Early Manifest Glaucoma Trial (EMGT) was a prospective, randomized study that assessed the role of IOP reduction on progression in newly diagnosed, previously untreated patients with early manifest open-angle glaucoma (OAG).[4] Progression of glaucoma was based on perimetric and photographic optic disc criteria. Patients excluded from the study included those with:

- Advanced visual field defects
- Visual acuity worse than 20/40
- Mean IOP >30 mm Hg
- Any IOP >35 mm Hg in at least one eye
- Any condition (eg, lens opacities) precluding reliable visual field or disc photography, use of study treatments, or 4-year follow-up.

After 6 years of follow-up, 53% of patients progressed. Based on multivariate analysis, the progression risk was reduced by 50% with treatment, and the risk of glaucoma progression was decreased by approximately 10% for each millimeter of mercury of initial IOP reduction. Predictive baseline factors for progression included higher baseline IOP, exfoliation, bilateral disease, worse static perimetric mean deviation, and older age. In addition, more frequent occurrence of optic disc hemorrhages during follow-up increased the risk of progression.

Normal-Pressure Glaucoma

Even when it is in the normal range, the level of IOP may play a significant role in the progression of visual defects among patients with normal-pressure glaucoma (NPG) or normal-tension glaucoma (NTG). The Collaborative Normal-Tension Glaucoma Study (CNTGS) was designed to determine whether IOP contributes to the progression of field loss in patients with

NPG. One eye of each of 140 eligible patients was selected for randomization to either the treatment arm or the control arm of the study. An IOP reduction of 30% from baseline was achieved for each eye in the treatment arm whereas each eye in the control arm was left untreated.[5] Among the control eyes, 35% showed definite progression of glaucomatous optic disc cupping or glaucomatous visual field loss compared with 12% of the treated eyes (P <0.0001). The study concluded that the level of IOP is involved in disease progression in patients with NPG as well as being implicated in its pathogenesis.

Risk of Blindness

A retrospective, cohort, case-control study compared patients who became legally blind from glaucoma with those who retained vision.[6] This community-based longitudinal study followed residents from Olmsted County, Minnesota—who were newly diagnosed with OAG between 1965 and 1980—through 1998. Fifty-six of 290 (19.3%) patients progressed to legal blindness in at least one eye over the 34-year period of the study. Of those patients who advanced to blindness, most already had moderate to advanced visual field loss at the time of diagnosis. An individual patient's susceptibility to IOP was demonstrated to be highly variable. Some patients with initially normal optic discs and visual fields became blind at IOP levels near 20 mm Hg, while others did not have any visual loss. Moreover, alterations in medical therapy (after progressive worsening of the visual field) were found less effective in lowering IOP in those becoming blind than in those not progressing to blindness.

The Olmstead County Study concluded that patients at greatest risk of blindness were those with initial visual field loss at the time of diagnosis and that some patients became blind at IOP levels that others tolerated without visual loss. The study investigators recommended that both continuous monitoring of visual fields and reassessment of target IOP levels in the setting of field progression be adopted as fundamental concepts in the long-term management of glaucoma.

REFERENCES

1. Leibowitz HM, Krueger DE, Maunder LR, et al. The Framingham Eye Study monograph: an ophthalmological and epidemiological study of cataract, glaucoma, diabetic retinopathy, macular degeneration, and visual acuity in a general population of 2631 adults, 1973-1975. *Surv Ophthalmol.* 1980;24(suppl):335-610.

2. Kass MA, Heuer DK, Higginbotham EJ, et al. The Ocular Hypertension Treatment Study: a randomized trial determines that topical ocular hypotensive medication delays or prevents the onset of primary open-angle glaucoma. *Arch Ophthalmol.* 2002;120:701-713.

3. Sommer A, Katz J, Quigley HA, et al. Clinically detectable nerve fiber atrophy precedes the onset of glaucomatous field loss. *Arch Ophthalmol.* 1991;109:77-83.

4. Leske MC, Heijl A, Hussein M, et al. Factors for glaucoma progression and the effect of treatment. The Early Manifest Glaucoma Trial. *Arch Ophthalmol.* 2003;121:48-56.

5. Collaborative Normal-Tension Glaucoma Study Group. Comparison of glaucomatous progression between untreated patients with normal-tension glaucoma and patients with therapeutically reduced intraocular pressures. *Am J Ophthalmol.* 1998;126:487-497.

6. Oliver JE, Hattenhauer MG, Herman D, et al. Blindness and glaucoma: a comparison of patients progressing to blindness from glaucoma with patients maintaining vision. *Am J Ophthalmol.* 2002;133:764-772.

7

Pitfalls in Diagnosis: Primary Open-Angle Glaucoma

Nonglaucomatous Optic Neuropathy

Although glaucoma is the most common cause of optic atrophy, it is important not to overlook other possible causes of optic atrophy even in the presence of elevated intraocular pressure (IOP). In glaucomatous optic atrophy, the cup typically enlarges before the area of pallor increases; this finding differs from that observed in nonglaucomatous causes of optic atrophy wherein the area of pallor is usually larger than that of the cup.[1] Thus the area of optic disc pallor should be carefully distinguished from the actual area of observed optic disc cupping in order to avoid misinterpretation of nonglaucomatous optic disc cupping.

Nerve fiber bundle visual field defects that are typical of glaucomatous optic neuropathy (GON) may also be caused by other diseases.[2] To help distinguish glaucomatous damage from other types of damage, the pattern of alterations (cupping) in the optic nerve should correspond to the appearance of the visual field defect. If there is not one-to-one correspondence, another source of the field defect should be sought. Conditions that might lead to nerve fiber bundle–associated visual field loss (and thereby mimic GON) are listed in **Table 7.1**.

A diagnosis of normal-pressure glaucoma (NPG) should be considered with caution. It is the most probable diagnosis only when the visual field defect(s) (nerve fiber bundle) and the optic atrophy (cupping) are both typical of glaucoma. If either the field

TABLE 7.1 — Nonglaucomatous Causes of Nerve Fiber Bundle–Associated Visual Field Defects

- Chorioretinitis
- Myopic retinal degeneration
- Optic nerve compressive lesions
- Optic nerve head drusen
- Optic nerve ischemia
- Optic neuritis
- Refractive scotoma
- Retinal laser damage
- Trauma

Adapted from Hoskins HD Jr, Kass MA. *Becker-Shaffer's Diagnosis and Therapy of the Glaucomas*. 6th ed. St. Louis, Mo: CV Mosby Co; 1989:151.

defect(s) or the optic atrophy are atypical, then it is essential to consider the gamut of differential diagnoses. In that connection, congenital colobomas can mimic glaucomatous optic disc cupping, and there may be associated visual field loss which can lead to a misdiagnosis of glaucoma.[3,4]

Abnormal Central Corneal Thickness

A significant number of eyes may have inaccurate readings of their IOP level, as measured by Goldmann applanation tonometry, because of the effects of central corneal thickness (CCT) on these measurements.[5] For a cornea with central thickness >600 microns, the true IOP may be significantly lower than the IOP value measured. Conversely, in eyes with CCT <500 microns, the true IOP may be much higher than that measured by Goldmann applanation tonometry. These effects may lead to an overdiagnosis or underdiagnosis of ocular hypertension and primary open-angle glaucoma (POAG). Consequently, in patients suspected of having glaucoma based on other signs, corneal pachymetry to determine CCT should be performed routinely to obtain a more accurate assessment of the IOP level.

Unilateral Glaucoma

Unilateral open-angle glaucoma (OAG) is usually due to:

- Pseudoexfoliation glaucoma
- Pigmentary (or pigment dispersion) glaucoma
- Steroid-induced glaucoma
- Glaucoma associated with trauma.

■ Exfoliation (Pseudoexfoliation) Glaucoma

Exfoliation syndrome is characterized by deposi-tions of fibrillar material in the anterior segment of the eye, including:

- Anterior lens surface and iris
- Zonules and ciliary processes
- Pigmentary abnormalities of the pupillary iris and trabecular meshwork
- Secondary open-angle glaucoma.[6]

Glaucoma associated with this syndrome is thought to be due to obstruction of aqueous flow through the tra-becular meshwork. This condition may be either uni-ocular or binocular, and the associated glaucoma is often unilateral with higher IOPs than that routinely observed in POAG.[7]

■ Pigmentary (or Pigment Dispersion) Glaucoma

The pigment dispersion syndrome (PDS) com-prises pigment deposition on the corneal endothelium in a vertical, spindlelike pattern (known as Kruken-berg's spindle), on the periphery of the lens, and in the trabecular meshwork.[7] PDS:

- Is usually bilateral
- Most often occurs in young, myopic white males
- May regress in later life.[8,9]

The mechanism of underlying PDS has been attributed to shedding of pigment from the posterior iris surface due to abrasion by anterior zonular packets with corresponding peripheral iris transillumination.[10] Phagocytosis of pigment by the trabecular meshwork may lead to collapse of the trabecular beams and, ultimately, to irreversible obstruction of aqueous outflow and elevated IOP.[11] Individuals with PDS have a 25% to 50% risk of developing open-angle glaucoma (OAG), which usually takes 15 to 20 years to develop.[12] Pigmentary glaucoma has been defined as PDS with IOP >21 mm Hg, with or without optic nerve damage or visual field loss. However, pigmentary glaucoma can also be defined as PDS with documented disc damage and visual field loss.[13]

■ Steroid-induced Glaucoma

Topical corticosteroids applied to the ocular and facial region may cause an increase in IOP that ranges from mild to severe. A similar type of response from systemic use of corticosteroids is also possible but less likely. The increased IOP may cause GON and may mimic POAG. In addition, patients with POAG are more susceptible to steroid-induced IOP elevation than patients without known glaucoma. Since elevated IOP may develop at any point during long-term topical steroid therapy, IOP needs to be monitored continuously in all patients during such treatment.[7]

■ Glaucoma Associated With Trauma

Unilateral OAG may result when the eye is subject to blunt or penetrating trauma that causes damage to the trabecular meshwork or leads to angle recession.[7] Any patient with a history of blunt ocular trauma, often with associated hyphema, should be examined by gonioscopy for an angle recession. Any patient with an angle recession should be followed regularly since the risk of developing glaucoma is still present even after 20 to 25 years. The greater the extent and severity of angle involvement, the greater the risk of glaucoma. Conversely, when a patient presents with unilateral glaucoma and a history of trauma, angle recession should be suspected.

Anterior Chamber Depth

Anterior chamber depth, specifically a shallow chamber, is a factor in the pathogenesis of primary angle-closure glaucoma (PACG).[14,15] Major asymmetry in anterior chamber depth between eyes is rare, but very small degrees of asymmetry are common in PACG.[15]

REFERENCES

1. Schwartz B. Cupping and pallor of the optic disc. *Arch Ophthalmol.* 1973;89:272-277.

2. Hoskins HD Jr, Kass MA. *Becker-Shaffer's Diagnosis and Therapy of the Glaucomas.* 6th ed. St. Louis, Mo: CV Mosby Co; 1989:151.

3. Jensen PE, Kalina RE. Congenital anomalies of the optic disc. *Am J Ophthalmol.* 1976;82:27-31.

4. Pagon RA. Ocular coloboma. *Surv Ophthalmol.* 1981;25:223-236.

5. Herndon L. Rethinking pachymetry and intraocular pressure. *Rev Ophthalmol.* 2002;July:88-90.

6. Naumann GO, Schlotzer-Schrehardt U, Kuchle M. Pseudo-exfoliation syndrome for the comprehensive ophthalmologist. Intraocular and systemic manifestations. *Ophthalmology.* 1998;105:951-968.

7. American Academy of Ophthalmology. *Glaucoma. Basic and Clinical Science Course 2003-2004.* San Francisco, Calif: American Academy of Ophthalmology; 2003:81-99.

8. Ritch R. Nonprogressive low-tension glaucoma with pigmentary dispersion. *Am J Ophthalmol.* 1982;94:190-196.

9. Speakman JS. Pigmentary dispersion. *Br J Ophthalmol.* 1981;65:249-251.

10. Campbell DG. Pigmentary dispersion and glaucoma. A new theory. *Arch Ophthalmol.* 1979;97:1667-1672.

11. Barton K. Secondary glaucomas: classification and management. In: Hitchings RA, ed. *Glaucoma.* London: BMJ Publishing Group; 2000:196-213.

12. Migliazzo CV, Shaffer RN, Nykin R, Magee S. Long-term analysis of pigmentary dispersion syndrome and pigmentary glaucoma. *Ophthalmology.* 1986;93:1528-1536.

13. Campbell DG, Schertzer RM. Pigmentary glaucoma. In: Ritch R, Shields MB, Krupin T, eds. *The Glaucomas.* 2nd ed. St. Louis, Mo: Mosby; 1996:801-819.

14. Tornquist R. Shallow anterior chamber is acute angle-closure. A clinical and genetic study. *Acta Ophthalmol.* 1953;31:1-74.

15. Ritch R, Lowe RF. Angle-closure glaucoma: mechanisms and epidemiology. In: Ritch R, Shields MB, Krupin T, eds. *The Glaucomas.* 2nd ed. St. Louis, Mo: Mosby; 1996:801-819.

8

Treatment Modalities: The Basis of Glaucoma Therapy

A number of landmark studies (Chapter 9, *Landmark Glaucoma Studies*) have firmly established the relationship between elevated intraocular pressure (IOP) and an increased risk of visual loss in patients with ocular hypertension (OH), primary open-angle glaucoma (POAG), and normal-pressure glaucoma (NPG).[1-4] At the present time, lowering IOP is the only proven method for slowing optic nerve damage and visual field loss progression.[5] Therapeutic options for lowering IOP involve either:

- Decreasing aqueous humor production
- Enhancing aqueous humor outflow.

The methods available to achieve either of these options include (**Table 8.1**):

- Medication
- Laser surgery
- Incisional surgery.

In the majority of cases, medications are used as first-line therapy for treating glaucoma. Although there may be greater long-term financial costs compared with surgery, pharmacologic treatment is often associated with decreased risks to the patient.[6]

Decreasing Aqueous Humor Production

■ Medication Therapy

Aqueous humor production occurs at the rate of about 2 to 2.5 microliters per minute.[7] There are sev-

TABLE 8.1 — SUMMARY OF MEDICAL AND SURGICAL METHODS FOR LOWERING INTRAOCULAR PRESSURE

Treatment Method	Decreasing Aqueous Humor Production	Increasing Aqueous Humor Outflow
Medication	• β-Blockers • Carbonic anhydrase inhibitors • Adrenergic agonists	• Cholinergic agonists • Prostaglandin derivatives • Adrenergic agonists
Laser surgery	• Cyclodestruction	• Trabeculoplasty
Incisional surgery	—	• Filtering surgery (trabeculectomy) • Shunt implants • Internal drainage (eg, viscocanulostomy)

eral classes of medications (eg, β-blockers, carbonic anhydrase inhibitors [CAIs], α-agonists) that lower IOP by decreasing aqueous humor production. Most of these agents are applied topically (**Table 8.2**). β-Adrenergic agonists and the carbonic anhydrase enzyme are both involved in the active secretion of aqueous humor. Thus β-adrenergic antagonists (β-blockers) and CAIs decrease aqueous humor production.[7] Since the introduction of timolol in the late 1970s, β-blockers have been the agents most widely used for lowering IOP.[8] Although highly effective in reducing IOP by as much as one third from baseline with few ocular side effects, β-blockers are also associated with systemic side effects that may be serious and some-

---

TABLE 8.2 — AQUEOUS INFLOW INHIBITORS

β-Blockers:
- Timolol
- Betaxolol
- Levobunolol
- Carteolol
- Metipranolol

Carbonic Anhydrase Inhibitors (CAIs):
- Systemic:
  - Acetazolamide
  - Methazolamide
  - Dichlorphenamide
- Topical:
  - Dorzolamide
  - Brinzolamide

Adrenergic Agonists:
- Nonspecific:
  - Epinephrine*
- $α_2$-Agonists:
  - Brimonidine†
  - Apraclonidine†

* Also increases conventional outflow.
† Also increases uveoscleral outflow.

times fatal. Previously, oral CAIs played an important role in the treatment of glaucoma. Poorly tolerated due to their high side-effect profile, they have been largely replaced by more recently developed topical forms that have fewer side effects.[8]

One manner by which α_2-adrenergic–receptor agonists are thought to lower IOP is by suppression of aqueous humor production.[6] When initially introduced as an IOP-lowering drug, the first of these medications was associated with systemic hypotension. Recently, newer selective α_2-agonists have been introduced that appear to have fewer effects on systemic blood pressure, but are associated with some ocular side effects.[8] Moreover, in patients with OH, brimonidine (a selective α_2-agonist) was found initially to induce IOP reduction with a decrease in aqueous humor production. However, after chronic treatment (29 days of treatment), the reduced IOP was associated with an increase in uveoscleral outflow only (the aqueous flow reversed back to baseline levels).[9]

■ Laser Surgery

Cyclodestruction is a surgical procedure by which aqueous production is decreased by damaging the ciliary processes (which secrete aqueous humor) as a means of lowering IOP. This procedure is often reserved for glaucomas that are refractory to standard medical and/or surgical therapy, such as neovascular or aphakic glaucoma.[10] The technique has evolved from diathermy (in the early 1930s) to cryotherapy, xenon arc photocoagulation, and finally to use of the Nd:YAG and semiconductor diode lasers for contact or noncontact transscleral cyclophotocoagulation. Although transscleral cyclodestruction has been utilized for many years, Nd:YAG and diode lasers have generated renewed interest in this modality. Ocular complications associated with cyclodestruction usually resolve with the use of topical steroids and cycloplegic agents. In best case scenarios, these laser procedures may lower IOP by as much as 44% to 68%.[11]

Increasing Aqueous Humor Outflow

Increasing aqueous humor outflow is another method for lowering IOP. Although decreasing aqueous production or increasing outflow can produce significant reductions in IOP, there are certain factors that render the latter a more physiological approach. Glaucoma is believed to result from increased resistance to aqueous outflow rather than a change in aqueous inflow.[12] Thus increasing outflow facility:

- Corrects the deficit that causes elevated IOP in glaucomatous eyes
- Protects against IOP spikes
- Helps to stabilize IOP levels
- Preserves the function of aqueous humor.

Medications that increase facility of outflow tend to be more effective in preventing pressure spikes and in maintaining IOP within a steady state range compared with those that reduce aqueous inflow. Because aqueous humor transports nutrients and other vital constituents to the avascular structures in the anterior chamber (ie, cornea and lens) while removing toxic metabolites, diminishing aqueous production may be deleterious to the eye.[13] Therefore, it may be advantageous to lower IOP by improving outflow as opposed to limiting production of aqueous humor.

Aqueous outflow follows both conventional and nonconventional pathways. The conventional pathway, which accounts for 83% to >90% of aqueous outflow, consists of the trabecular meshwork, Schlemm's canal, intrascleral channels, and episcleral and conjunctival veins.[11] Although the nonconventional pathway may involve a number of routes for the outflow of aqueous humor, its principal route is via the uveal tract and sclera: hence the term uveoscleral outflow. Earlier studies suggested that this pathway accounted for only 10% to 15% of total outflow.[14] However, more recent investigations suggest that the uveoscleral pathway may reach as high as 40% to 50%.[15] With regard to this discrepancy, it should be noted that current methods of measuring uveoscleral outflow in humans are subject to multiple sources of error, and therefore yield nothing more than estimated values.[16]

Whereas conventional outflow is dependent on the baseline level of IOP, the nonconventional pathway is generally considered to be pressure independent.[17] IOP reduction can be achieved by enhancement of either conventional or nonconventional outflow or both. In patients with glaucoma due to blockage of the conventional pathway, it may be feasible to alter uveoscleral outflow sufficiently to reduce and even normalize IOP. A number of topical ocular hypotensive medications increase aqueous humor outflow (**Table 8.3**).

TABLE 8.3 — AQUEOUS OUTFLOW ENHANCERS
Conventional/Trabecular:
• Cholinergic agonists (parasympathomimetics):   – Pilocarpine   – Echothiophate iodide   – Carbachol   • Prostaglandin derivatives: – Bimatoprost   – Latanoprost   • Nonspecific adrenergic agonists: – Epinephrine
Nonconventional/Uveoscleral:
• Prostaglandin derivatives: – Latanoprost   – Bimatoprost   – Travoprost   – Unoprostone   • α_2-Agonists: – Brimonidine

■ Medical Enhancement of Conventional Outflow

There are relatively few classes of topical ocular drugs whose primary mechanism of action is to increase conventional aqueous humor outflow. This IOP-lowering method is desirable given its ability to offset the IOP spikes to which glaucoma patients are especially vulnerable. Cholinergic stimulators (parasympathomimetics), such as the miotics pilocarpine and echothiophate iodide, enhance conventional/trabecular outflow.[18] However, miotic agents are associated with multiple ocular and systemic side effects that limit their utility, and pilocarpine has the added disadvantage of suppressing uveoscleral outflow.

Although not the predominant mechanism by which prostaglandin (PG) derivatives lower IOP, some studies have reported that latanoprost and bimatoprost also enhance trabecular outflow. In particular, latanoprost and bimatoprost were found to increase tonographic outflow facility in normal volunteers, and latanoprost was also found to increase outflow facility in OH.[12,19]

Nonspecific adrenergic agonists (sympathomimetics), such as epinephrine, have a dual action in that they initially reduce aqueous production and then enhance conventional outflow. In the past, epinephrine was a standard agent for lowering IOP, although it is less often used today due to its extraocular, intraocular, and systemic side effects.[20]

■ Medical Enhancement of Nonconventional Outflow

Adrenergic agonists, including α_2-agonists (eg, brimonidine), may increase nonconventional outflow in addition to their primary action, decreasing aqueous humor production. In contrast, the primary means by which PG derivatives lower IOP is via increasing uveoscleral outflow.[21-24] The PG analogues include:

- Latanoprost

85

- Bimatoprost
- Travoprost
- Unoprostone

■ Laser Surgery—Trabeculoplasty

Early attempts at reducing IOP involved using a laser to create holes in the trabecular meshwork to improve aqueous outflow.[25,26] However, these openings eventually closed, with a resultant increase in IOP. Long-term successful lowering of IOP was eventually achieved by placing evenly spaced, low-energy, nonpenetrating laser burns around a portion of or the entire circumference of the trabecular meshwork.[27] This technique, laser trabeculoplasty (LTP), increases facility of outflow, thereby reducing IOP by about 20% from baseline. Most of the experience with LTP has been gained using the argon laser. The IOP-lowering effect of argon laser trabeculoplasty (ALT) is maintained in approximately:

- 70% to 80% of eyes for 1 year
- 35% to 50% of eyes after 5 years
- 20% to 30% of eyes at 10 years.[28]

ALT is indicated in patients whose glaucoma is inadequately controlled by medications, and may be indicated prior to proceeding with glaucoma filtration and/or cataract-lens implant surgery.[28]

Selective laser trabeculoplasty (SLT) was developed to produce the beneficial effect on conventional outflow facility associated with ALT without causing scarring and destruction of the trabecular meshwork due to thermal coagulation. SLT is performed with a frequency-doubled Nd:YAG laser (532 nanometer wavelength) that is Q-switched to emit a pulsed beam of 3 nanoseconds duration (400 micron spot size).[29,30] In practice, SLT places 50 contiguous non-overlapping spots around 180° of trabecular circumference at an approximate energy level of 0.8 mJ. There is said to be no collateral thermal damage because of the low spatial concentration of energy at the treatment site (approximately 0.002 mJ per micron for SLT vs 0.8 mJ per micron for ALT), and rapid pulse duration below the thermal relaxation time of the melanin target.

SLT is reported to yield a decrease in IOP similar to that of ALT.[29,31] In the absence of coagulative damage, trabecular structure is preserved. SLT, unlike ALT, has the theoretical advantage of repeatability when the initial beneficial effect has dissipated. If these preliminary results are confirmed, then SLT might be deployed as first-line treatment for POAG. In addition, SLT may be effective in eyes that previously underwent ALT. While promising, SLT requires more long-term clinical studies of efficacy and safety before it can be recommended as the preferred method of LTP.

■ External Drainage to Enhance Outflow

Surgical techniques are used to bypass the normal outflow system. The most common incisional procedure for glaucoma is penetrating filtration surgery. In all filtration surgeries, an opening or fistula is created at the limbus to allow aqueous humor to drain from the anterior chamber. In this manner, any obstructions to outflow are bypassed, and aqueous humor passes into the subconjunctival space, thereby forming a filtering bleb. The aqueous fluid then leaves the bleb by means of several drainage routes (eg, transconjunctival flow).[32]

Filtration surgery can be comprised of either full-thickness or guarded techniques. Because full-thickness or unguarded filtration procedures are associated with a number of complications due to excessive drainage of aqueous humor, they have given way to partial-thickness or guarded procedures. Trabeculectomy *ab externo* is the most commonly performed guarded filtration procedure. Although the original intent of trabeculectomy was to facilitate drainage into Schlemm's canal, the resultant decreased IOP was found to occur primarily via external filtration with formation of sub-conjunctival filtering blebs.[33,34]

An alternative to trabeculectomy surgery involves the placement of aqueous shunt implants. Glaucoma tube shunts are often utilized in patients with poor prognoses for achieving successful outcomes with conventional glaucoma filtration surgery. The posterior implant design utilizes a tube in the anterior chamber or vitreous cavity to shunt ocular fluid to a posteriorly placed external plate reservoir (ie, explant).[35] The episcleral fluid reservoir is usually delineated by fibrous encapsulation that develops around the explant.

Common shunt devices employed include the Baerveldt implant with its open tube design or the Ahmed implant with its restrictive tube design.[36] Various modifications have been described to disable initially the aqueous flow through the open Baerveldt tube (eg, ripcord stent technique, dissolvable ligature suture technique, etc) in an attempt to decrease the incidence of postoperative complications associated with hypotony.[37] In contrast, the Ahmed tube implant contains a pressure-regulating valve to help prevent excessive drainage of aqueous fluid.

In a recent publication, Tsai and colleagues reported the results of a single surgeon comparison of surgical outcomes of Ahmed and Baerveldt shunt implants in the treatment of refractory glaucoma.[38] Survival curve analysis showed similar success rates between the two patient groups up to 2 years postoperatively (**Figure 8.1**). The Ahmed group exhibited lower IOPs in the immediate postoperative period (ie, up to 1 week) and took fewer glaucoma medications at 1 week and 1 month postsurgery. However, there was a higher prevalence and earlier onset of bleb encapsulation observed with the Ahmed shunt. There was also a nonsignificant tendency toward higher occurrence of choroidal effusions with the Baerveldt implant.

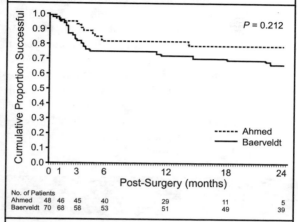

FIGURE 8.1 — AHMED VS BAERVELDT SHUNT IMPLANTS IN THE TREATMENT OF REFRACTORY GLAUCOMA

Cumulative probability of success for the Ahmed *(dotted line)* and Baerveldt *(solid line)* groups.

Modified from: Tsai JC, et al. *Ophthalmology.* 2003;110:1814-1821.

■ Internal Drainage to Enhance Outflow

Types of nonpenetrating filtration surgery (NPFS) that depend on internal drainage include:

- Viscocanalostomy
- Deep sclerectomy.

These procedures involve excision of an inner scleral flap that extends down to Descemet's membrane and then unroofing of the canal of Schlemm without actual penetration into the interior of the eye. They allow aqueous humor to exit the anterior chamber by seeping through a thin, almost transparent, Descemet's-trabecular membrane into a surgically created subscleral lake.[39] Having bypassed the glaucomatous trabecular obstruction, fluid then passes into the unroofed

89

Schlemm's canal and leaves the eye via normal internal drainage channels. Due to this subscleral-canalicular outflow pathway, subconjunctival filtration with bleb formation is minimal, and often not observed. Hence, bleb-related complications are minimized.

Although NPFS procedures have some theoretical advantages over trabeculectomy (eg, fewer perioperative restrictions and decreased likelihood of hypotony-related complications), disadvantages include a lesser degree of IOP reduction following surgery, and an increased reliance on surgical skill for successful execution and outcome. Moreover, investigators have yet to determine the long-term success and safety of NPFS procedures.

General Considerations for Medication Treatment

■ **Efficacy of a Drug to Achieve Desired Reduction in Intraocular Pressure**

The selection of a target IOP (to be discussed in the next section, *Setting Target Pressures*) is achieved by choosing either a percentage reduction or an actual IOP value or range. However, there is a lack of consensus regarding the accuracy and calculation of either method. Nevertheless, once a target IOP level has been calculated, suitable medication(s) must then be selected to achieve the desired goal. The questions that a clinician must ask are:

- How much should the baseline IOP be lowered (either by percentage reduction or to achieve a target IOP value)?
- Is the resultant level of pressure reduction sufficient to control the glaucoma in that particular patient?
- Is it necessary to add or switch to additional agents to achieve the target pressure (which may

unnecessarily compromise patient safety and medication compliance)?

■ Controlling Diurnal Variations in Intraocular Pressure

The ability of a topical hypotensive agent to control diurnal variations in IOP is highly desirable. In patients with POAG or OH, IOP and aqueous flow are known to follow the day-type circadian curve such that IOP peaks in the morning (between 8 AM and 10 AM) and reaches a trough level at night.[40] However, this day-type IOP curve was not observed in both young (18 to 25 years of age) and older (50 to 69 years of age) healthy volunteers who exhibited nocturnal elevation of IOP (**Figure 8**.2).[41] The trough IOP level was measured at the end of the light/wake period while the peak IOP appeared at the beginning of the dark period. The nocturnal IOP elevation was largely explained by the shift from daytime upright posture to nighttime supine posture.

Asrani and colleagues have demonstrated that large diurnal fluctuations in IOP (as measured by home tonometry) create significant risk factors for disease progression in patients with open-angle glaucoma (OAG).[42] In their study's 8-year follow-up period, 88% of patients with the highest 25th percentile of IOP fluctuation had disease progression, compared with only 57% of patients in the lowest 25th percentile of IOP fluctuation. Orzalesi and coworkers have shown that PG derivatives, such as latanoprost, yield a relatively flat diurnal IOP curve by providing a fairly uniform circadian reduction in IOP.[40] In contrast, timolol was less effective at reducing nocturnal IOP. Dorzolamide was less effective than latanoprost but still produced a significant reduction in nocturnal IOP.

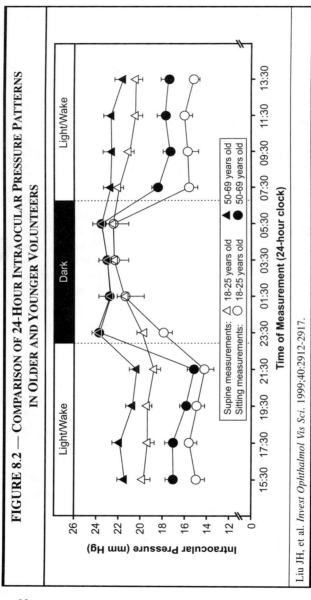

FIGURE 8.2 — COMPARISON OF 24-HOUR INTRAOCULAR PRESSURE PATTERNS IN OLDER AND YOUNGER VOLUNTEERS

Liu JH, et al. *Invest Ophthalmol Vis Sci.* 1999;40:2912-2917.

■ Efficacy at Trough Drug Concentrations

With regard to controlling diurnal variations in IOP, it is important to consider the trough IOP effects of topical hypotensive medications. When a pharmacologic agent provides adequate IOP reduction at trough concentration, it is assumed that its efficacy is sufficient at other times throughout the dosing cycle. This is especially relevant for drugs that are given once a day as monotherapy.[43] Latanoprost dosed once daily has an IOP-lowering effect that is fairly constant during the 24-hour circadian cycle.[44] Therapeutic strategies that are primarily based on β-blockers may offer less nocturnal protection since aqueous flow is already reduced at night and its baseline rate cannot be further suppressed. As noted in the Asrani study above,[42] the magnitude of diurnal variations in IOP may be more significant than absolute IOP values with regard to the development of glaucomatous optic neuropathy (GON). Thus, the extent of IOP reduction at a drug's trough concentration must be considered when choosing a specific medical regimen for glaucoma.

■ Balancing Efficacy and Tolerability

When considering topical hypotensive therapy, it is also necessary to balance efficacy against tolerability. These factors must be weighed on an individual basis since tolerability varies greatly from patient to patient. Certain agents, such as pilocarpine, yield significant reductions in IOPs, but have considerable side effects that impact medication compliance and a patient's willingness to continue therapy. In this regard, the therapeutic index (the ratio of a drug's efficacy to its side effects profile) needs to be factored into the choice of each medication. Drugs with a higher therapeutic index (ie, favorable ratio of efficacy to side effects) are preferred.

Clinicians need to also consider not just tolerability in general but the balance between local and systemic side effects. Certain classes of agents that include β-blockers and CAIs are associated with considerable and often serious systemic side effects. In contrast, PG derivatives are relatively free of systemic effects but have been associated with adverse ocular and visual effects. (The efficacy and side effects profiles of these agents will be addressed in Chapter 10, *Medications for Glaucoma*.) The degree to which patients are subjected to risks of systemic or ocular side effects will depend on the actual goal for IOP reduction. The target IOP level itself depends on the extent of GON and the risk of vision loss in a given patient. Safety and tolerability may be overriding priorities for patients who have mild or suspect disease. For patients with advanced disease and impending risk of serious visual loss, the physician and patient may choose to tolerate a greater degree of side effects to achieve an aggressive target IOP reduction with a more effective medical regimen.

■ Safety of Treatment Options

Medication, laser surgery, and incisional surgery are all options when treating glaucoma, although pharmacologic therapy is usually chosen as first-line treatment. However, filtration surgery and/or LTP may be considered when the severity and/or type of glaucoma is unlikely to respond favorably to medications. Obviously, the relative risks and benefits of each treatment modality must be assessed when selecting one over the other.

A direct comparison of the benefits of surgery vs medication was undertaken by the Collaborative Initial Glaucoma Treatment Study (CIGTS).[45,46] In this study, patients were randomized to either filtration surgery (trabeculectomy) or medication as initial therapy. After a 4-year follow-up period, CITGS demonstrated that visual field loss did not differ significantly between the two treatment modalities. In the early postoperative period, patients in the surgery group had a greater risk of substantial visual acuity loss compared with those in the medication group. The rate of cataract removal was also greater for the surgical group. At the end of 4 years, however, the average visual acuity in both groups was comparable. Mean IOP in the surgical group was 3 to 4 mm Hg lower than that for the medication group. CITGS concluded that aggressive treatment to lower IOP by both modalities resulted in minimal visual field loss over a 5-year period.

For chronic diseases such as POAG, a 4- to 5-year study period may not be of sufficient duration to warrant altering current treatment practices. It should be noted, however, that glaucoma surgery has a risk of substantial complications ranging from hemorrhage, hypotony, and lens opacities to loss of vision (**Table 8.4**). Although medication treatment is also associated with both systemic and ocular side effects, the use of newer therapeutic agents, such as the PG analogues, minimizes the risk of systemic side effects (although ocular and visual side effects do remain).

- ■ **Combining Medical Therapies—Additive or Synergistic Mechanisms of Action**

When elevated IOP remains refractory to a specific medication or is not reduced to a chosen target level, a common practice is to add other classes of ocular hypotensive agents to the initially chosen drug. Maximum tolerable medical therapy refers to concurrent deployment of as many agents with different mechanisms of action as proven to be additive in combination without producing intolerable side effects (**Table 8.5**). In practice, this combination represents a balance between efficacy, tolerability, and compliance for each individual patient. It rarely consists of more than three or perhaps four medications, and for certain patients may be no more than one or even zero. Such aggressive combination therapy may reduce IOP

TABLE 8.4 — COMPLICATIONS ASSOCIATED WITH INCISIONAL GLAUCOMA SURGERY AND ARGON LASER TRABECULOPLASTY

Incisional Glaucoma Surgery:
- Hemorrhage
- Inflammation
- Hypotony
- Shallow anterior chamber
- Malignant glaucoma
- Uveal effusion
- Lens opacities and cataract
- Endophthalmitis
- Visual loss

Argon Laser Trabeculoplasty:
- Elevated intraocular pressure
- Progressive visual field loss
- Peripheral anterior synechiae
- Iritis
- Hemorrhage
- Corneal abrasion
- Corneal edema and endothelial burns
- Syncope-vasovagal response

Adapted from: Bechetoille A, Hitchings RA. Glaucoma surgery. In: Hitchings RA, ed. *Glaucoma*. London: BMJ Publishing Group; 2000:91-105; and Weinreb RN. Laser trabeculoplasty. In: Ritch R, Shields MB, Krupin T, eds. *The Glaucomas*. 2nd ed. St. Louis, Mo: Mosby; 1996:1575-1590.

TABLE 8.5 — SUMMARY OF CRITERIA FOR SELECTING A SPECIFIC MEDICAL THERAPY

- Efficacy in achieving target IOP reduction
- Ability to control diurnal variations in IOP
- Efficacy at trough drug concentrations
- Efficacy vs tolerability—do benefits of drug outweigh risks of adverse effects?
- Comparative safety of agents
- Ease of use/dosing schedule
- Cost of medication

by as much as 40%,[43,45,47] and it may be initiated before advancing to LTP or incisional surgery.

Since β-blockers have been considered as primary therapy for glaucoma in the past, adjunctive therapy has usually consisted of adding a second-line agent to timolol, the most commonly used β-blocker. Almost all classes of ocular hypotensive medications have been paired with β-blockers to produce additive effects in lowering IOP. Maximum tolerable medical therapy may consist of several classes of medications, some in fixed combinations (**Table 8.6**).[6] The most logical fixed combination would be achieved by pairing an agent that increases aqueous outflow (to protect against pressure spikes) with a β-blocker that reduces aqueous production. In practice, the PG derivative, latanoprost, which increases uveoscleral outflow, is frequently prescribed in conjunction with timolol to produce an optimal reduction in IOP (see Chapter 10, *Medications for Glaucoma*).

8

■ Patient Compliance/Adherence to Medication Therapy

Adherence to topical glaucoma regimens is critical for maintaining sustained and consistent reduction

TABLE 8.6 — CLASSES OF TOPICAL HYPOTENSIVES USED IN COMBINATION THERAPY
Classes of Agents Commonly Used in Maximum-Tolerated Medical Therapy: • β-Blockers   • Prostaglandin derivatives   • Cholinergic agonists   • α-Agonists   • Carbonic anhydrase inhibitors (CAIs)
Combinations Under Current Use: • β-Blocker + CAI (timolol + dorzolamide [Cosopt])*
* Fixed combination.

of IOP. It has been estimated that noncompliance accounts for approximately 10% of visual loss in glaucoma, and is a leading cause of glaucoma blindness. There are multiple potential causes of noncompliance. Instillation of eyedrops requires some degree of skill and may be especially problematic for the elderly. Compliance is more likely to be compromised as the number of medications and complexity of the regimen increases. With multiple agents, there is increased dosing frequency, more lifestyle disruptions, and greater risk of side effects.

Recently Tsai and colleagues identified and described systematically the common obstacles to medication adherence (ie, compliance) as reported by patients with glaucoma.[48] Seventy-one unique situational obstacles were reported and grouped into four separate categories: situational/environmental factors (49%), medication regimen (32%), patient factors (16%), and provider factors (3%). **Table 8.7** presents a list of these situational obstacles to medication adherence. Utilization of this systematic classification of compliance barriers will assist in optimizing patient care by means of improved patient education and appropriate individualized selection of therapeutic regimens.

Claxton and colleagues reported that optimum medication compliance is achieved with less frequent dosing, and that compliance is inversely related to the complexity of the regimen across all therapeutic classes.[49] Patel and Spaeth found that almost 60% of patients failed to use eyedrops as prescribed.[50] They determined that significant factors affecting compliance were:

- Daily dose frequency
- Forgetfulness
- Inconvenience
- Reduced affordability of the medications.

Medication side effects and age did not appear to be significant factors for noncompliance in their study.[50] Other important factors for noncompliance include dissatisfaction with treatment, a misunderstanding of the disease, and the asymptomatic and chronic nature of the disease (generally without noticeable subjective improvement related to treatment). Procedures for optimizing compliance are listed in **Table 8.8**.

Patients who are often noncompliant with their regimen have been reported to demonstrate improved compliance immediately prior to a regularly scheduled office visit. Although progressive visual field loss was detected at the visit (as a result of noncompliance), their examination revealed stable and controlled IOP readings.[51] Since patients often do not admit to medication nonadherence, clinicians may wrongly assume that the maximum efficacy of the prescribed drug has been elicited and therefore proceed to increase medical therapy with more frequent dosing, greater drug concentrations, or additional medications.[52] Unless nonadherence to the glaucoma regimen is suspected or techniques to assess compliance are used, it is difficult to determine whether disease progression is due to lack of drug efficacy, medication tachyphylaxis, or patient noncompliance. This may be particularly relevant in the case of initial β-blocker therapy in which approximately 50% of patients need either medication substitution or addition after 2 years.[53]

Setting Target Pressures

A number of landmark studies—some of which will be described in Chapter 10, *Medications for Glaucoma*—have clearly demonstrated that aggressive lowering of IOP either slows or aborts the progression of optic nerve damage and visual field loss in glaucoma patients. For this reason, all types of glaucomas are treated by lowering IOP through medical therapy, la-

TABLE 8.7 — SITUATIONAL OBSTACLES TO MEDICATION COMPLIANCE/ADHERENCE IN PATIENTS WITH GLAUCOMA

Factor	Sample Statement
Regimen Factors	
Refill	I only forget to take my drops when I run out
Cost	When my insurance stopped paying for my medication, I didn't take my drops
Complexity	It was harder when I was taking four medications; now that I am taking three, it is better
Change	When I first started taking the drops, I had a harder time remembering
Side effects	I decided to quit taking my drops because I had a bad reaction from them
Patient Factors	
Knowledge/skill	Sometimes I miss my eye when taking my drops
Memory	Sometimes I just forget to take my drops
Motivation/health beliefs	I quit taking my drops because I didn't see benefit from them and didn't think they were working
Comorbidity	It is harder to keep track of my drops because I am taking so many other medications

Provider Factors	
Dissatisfaction	I quit taking my drops because I was dissatisfied with my doctor's care
Communication	I stopped taking my drops because I didn't understand initially that I need to take them forever
Situational/Environmental Factors	
Accountability/lack of support	Living alone, I had problems taking my drops; now I live with my daughter and have no problems
Major life events	Two years ago when my wife died, I had a hard time taking my drops
Travel/away from home	When I am on vacation, it is more difficult to take my drops
Competing activities	I miss my drops on Sunday morning when I go to church
Change in routine	Lifestyle changes that occur on weekends, such as not getting up at a normal hour, cause me to forget to take my drops

Tsai JC, et al. *J Glaucoma.* 2003;12:393-398.

TABLE 8.8 — PROCEDURES FOR OPTIMIZING PATIENT COMPLIANCE/ADHERENCE TO MEDICATIONS

- Minimize inconvenience—fit dosing schedule to patient's daily routine
- Teach instillation techniques
- Use compliance caps on medication bottles
- Use instillation frames
- Minimize number of drugs and dosing frequency
- Discuss nature of glaucoma and its treatment
- Alert patients to side effects
- Enhance patient communication and support

Adapted from: Goldberg I. Compliance. In: Ritch R, Shields MB, Krupin T, eds. *The Glaucomas*. 2nd ed. St. Louis, Mo: Mosby; 1996:1375-1384.

ser procedures, surgical methods, or a combination of the three. The goal of therapy is to achieve a range of IOP that will prevent or slow further damage and visual field loss. The upper boundary of this range is considered the target pressure. It will vary from patient to patient based on the individual severity of the disease. There may also be intrapatient variation in the target pressure needed to maintain vision over the long-term course of the disease.[54]

It is recommended that the initial target pressure should represent a numerical reduction of 20% to 30% from the pretreatment IOP level assumed to have contributed to disease progression. The severity of disease can be determined by a comprehensive examination that evaluates, among other factors, the status of the optic nerve head, fundus, and retinal nerve fiber layer, as well as the degree of visual field loss. An initial target IOP lowering of as much as 40% may be sought based on the severity of disease (mild, moderate, or severe) and the presence of other risk factors such as:

- Family history
- Genetic susceptibility

- Age
- Race
- Ethnic factors
- Refractive errors.

One treatment algorithm established by the Preferred Practice Pattern Committee (Glaucoma Panel) of the American Academy of Ophthalmology calls for an initial reduction in IOP of 20% to 30%. When the target level is achieved but disease progression continues, the panel suggests that a further pressure lowering of >15% should be sought.[54]

Essentially, the more advanced the disease, the lower the initial target pressure must be set. This numerical goal is a best estimate, since there is currently no means of determining the absolute cutoff pressure that will prevent further glaucomatous damage.[54] However, the greater and more consistent the IOP reduction, the greater the decrease in risk for further GON. As noted earlier, IOP lowering is still the only proven option for halting progression of glaucoma.[6] One means of determining a specific individual's target pressure level is to obtain documentation of disease progression in its earlier stages and to assess the rate of progression since then. This information may serve as a guide for determining the appropriate aggressiveness of IOP-lowering therapy. In establishing an individual target range, diurnal IOP variation with its associated night time peaks must also be taken into account.

Target IOP may be set either as an absolute number or as a percentage reduction from the pretreatment baseline pressure. An argument for absolute values was provided by the Advanced Glaucoma Intervention Study (AGIS), which found that pressures <18 mm Hg were more effective in slowing progression of visual field loss compared with IOPs >18 mm Hg.[2] However, the various clinical factors associated with a specific patient should drive the selection of a target IOP range rather than simple reliance on absolute IOP value(s) based on arbitrary benchmarks.

By lowering IOP to the target range, the clinician seeks to stop, or at least retard, the rate of retinal ganglion cell (RGC) death, which varies widely among patients with POAG. To achieve this goal, it has been suggested that the targeted IOP lowering for mild, moderate, or severe glaucoma should be shifted upward to 30%, 40%, or 50%, respectively, from baseline IOP values. More aggressive therapy should be utilized when there is greater risk of GON and subsequent visual field loss.[55] This guideline may be used to determine the acceptable level of risk or adverse effects associated with the selection of specific anti-glaucoma therapies.

Another factor used to determine the appropriate aggressiveness of therapy is the patient's age. The patient's life expectancy should be weighed against an estimate of the rate and extent of RGC death. For each individual, a specific level of IOP is associated with a particular rate of RGC death. The visual effects associated with the RGC death rate (including the ability of the patient to retain useful central vision) depend to a great extent on the individual's life expectancy. Thus younger patients may need to be treated more aggressively than older patients (whose overall vision may not be significantly compromised during their remaining shorter life span).[56] However, it is almost impossible to predict both the rate of RGC loss and the life expectancy for a given patient. Moreover, older patients may also require aggressive IOP-lowering treatment since older age was a predictive risk factor for glaucomatous progression in the Early Manifest Glaucoma Trial (EMGT).[57] Older patients also may have a lower threshold of tolerability for the side effects associated with particular medications.

Unilateral Trials

To determine the efficacy of a chosen topical ocular antihypertensive agent, a unilateral therapeutic trial should be initiated. For this procedure to be valid, both the trial eye and the control eye must have similar IOP values (or a consistent ratio between them), and their diurnal and long-term IOP fluctuations should be similar as well.[58] By treating one eye and observing the other as a control, the clinician is able to assess the efficacy of the IOP-lowering agent. In doing so, the medication may be discontinued if it is found to be:

- Ineffective
- Inconvenient to use
- The cause of undue side effects.[59]

When bilateral therapy is assumed to be ineffective, a reverse unilateral trial can also be performed in which an agent is discontinued in one eye only. This reverse trial may also unmask diurnal swings in IOP in the untreated experimental eye, thereby confirming the efficacy of the discontinued drug.

Reducing Systemic Absorption of Topical Medications

Topically-instilled glaucoma medications exert their desired IOP-lowering effect by penetrating through the cornea to gain access to targeted intraocular receptor sites. Undesired systemic side effects of these topical agents result from their access to non-ocular sites via alternate pathways. One pathway is via tear flow into the lacrimal drainage system and through a surface of highly vascular nasopharygeal mucosa, thereby leading to absorption into the bloodstream without prior passage through the liver. Although this alternate pathway can result in adverse reactions (in susceptible individuals) from any of the glaucoma medications, β-blocker agents and α-adrenergic agonists are major offenders in terms of frequency and severity of such complications.

Significant reduction of tear flow into the lacrimal drainage system can be achieved by digital nasolacrimal occlusion or even by simple eyelid closure alone, which stops the nasolacrimal pump mechanism. In a study involving normal volunteers, it was shown that either nasolacrimal occlusion or eyelid closure for five minutes (after topical instillation of timolol 0.5%) reduced the resultant serum concentration of the drug by more than 60%.[60] Moreover, these same maneuvers increased the aqueous humor concentration of topically-instilled fluorescein, presumably because of prolonged contact with the cornea. In practice, nasolacrimal occlusion and/or eyelid closure is recommended for approximately 3 minutes to facilitate compliance and enhance the therapeutic index. In special situations where a systemically-intolerable agent would otherwise be of considerable benefit (such as averting unwanted surgical intervention), the clinician might consider cautious resumption of that agent after insertion of a lower punctal plug in one or both eyes as needed.[61]

REFERENCES

1. Kass MA, Heuer DK, Higginbotham EJ, et al. The Ocular Hypertension Treatment Study: a randomized trial determines that topical ocular hypotensive medication delays or prevents the onset of primary open-angle glaucoma. *Arch Ophthalmol.* 2002;120:701-713.

2. The AGIS Investigators. The Advanced Glaucoma Intervention Study (AGIS) 7: the relationship between control of intraocular pressure and visual field deterioration. *Am J Ophthalmol.* 2000;130:429-440.

3. Collaborative Normal-Tension Glaucoma Study Group. Comparison of glaucomatous progression between untreated patients with normal-tension glaucoma and patients with therapeutically reduced intraocular pressures. *Am J Ophthalmol.* 1998;126:487-497.

4. Collaborative Normal-Tension Glaucoma Study Group. The effectiveness of intraocular pressure reduction in the treatment of normal-tension glaucoma. *Am J Ophthalmol.* 1998;126:498-505.

5. Wax MB, Camras CB, Fiscella RG, Girkin C, Singh K, Weinreb RN. Emerging perspectives on glaucoma: optimizing 24-hr control of intraocular pressure. *Am J Ophthalmol.* 2002;133(suppl):S1-S10.

6. Choplin NT. Advances in the medical management of glaucoma. In: American Academy of Ophthalmology, ed. *A LEO Clinical Update Course on Glaucoma.* San Francisco, Calif: American Academy of Ophthalmology; 2000:1-8.

7. Brubaker RF. The flow of aqueous humor in the human eye. *Trans Am Ophthalmol Soc.* 1982;80:391-474.

8. Alward WL. Medical management of glaucoma. *N Engl J Med.* 1998;339:1298-1307.

9. Toris CB, Camras CB, Yablonski ME. Acute versus chronic effects of brimonidine on aqueous humor dynamics in ocular hypertensive patients. *Am J Ophthalmol.* 1999;128:8-14.

8

10. Schuman JS. Cyclodestruction. In: Epstein DL, Allingham RR, Schuman JS, eds. *Chandler and Grant's Glaucoma*. 4th ed. Baltimore, Md: Lippincott, Williams and Wilkins; 1997:484-485.

11. Stewart WC, Brindley GO, Shields MB. Cyclodestructive procedures. In: Ritch R, Shields MB, Krupin T, eds. *Glaucomas*. 2nd ed. St. Louis, Mo: Mosby-Year Book; 1996: 1605-1630.

12. Brubaker RF. Mechanism of action of bimatoprost (Lumigan). *Surv Ophthalmol*. 2001;45(suppl 4):S347-S351.

13. Shields MB. *Textbook of Glaucoma*. 4th ed. Baltimore, Md: Lippincott, Williams and Wilkins; 1998:12.

14. Epstein DL. Practical aqueous humor dynamics. In: Epstein DL, Allingham RR, Schuman JS, eds. *Chandler and Grant's Glaucoma*. 4th ed. Baltimore, Md: Lippincott, Williams and Wilkins; 1997:18-24.

15. Toris CB, Yablonski ME, Wang YL, Camras CB. Aqueous humor dynamics in the aging human eye. *Am J Ophthalmol*. 1999;127:407-412.

16. Brubaker RF. Measurement of uveoscleral outflow in humans. *J Glaucoma*. 2001;10(suppl 1):S45-S48.

17. van Buskirk EM. Anatomy. In: Epstein DL, Allingham RR, Schuman JS, eds. *Chandler and Grant's Glaucoma*. 4th ed. Baltimore, Md: Lippincott, Williams and Wilkins; 1997:6-17.

18. Shields MB. *Textbook of Glaucoma*. 4th ed. Baltimore, Md: Lippincott, Williams and Wilkins; 1998:384-397.

19. Ziai N, Dolan JW, Kacere RD, Brubaker RF. The effects on aqueous dynamics of PhXA41, a new prostaglandin F_2 alpha analogue, after topical application in normal and ocular hypertensive human eyes. *Arch Ophthalmol*. 1993;111:1351-1358.

20. Shields MB. *Textbook of Glaucoma*. 4th ed. Baltimore, Md: Williams and Wilkins; 1998:398, 402.

21. Watson PG. Latanoprost. Two years' experience of its use in the United Kingdom. Latanoprost Study Group. *Ophthalmology*. 1998;105:82-87.

22. Watson P, Stjernschantz J. A six month randomized double-masked study comparing latanoprost with timolol in open-angle glaucoma and ocular hypertension. The Latanoprost Study Group. *Ophthalmology*. 1996;103:126-137.

23. Toris CB, Camras C, Yablonski ME, Brubaker RF. Effects of exogenous prostaglandins on aqueous humor dynamics and blood-aqueous barrier function. *Surv Ophthalmol*. 1997;41(suppl 2):S69-S75.

24. Resul B, Stjernschantz J, Selen G, Bito L. Structure-activity relationships and receptor profiles of some ocular hypotensive prostanoids. *Surv Ophthalmol*. 1997;41(suppl 2):S47-S52.

25. Worthen DM, Wickham MG. Argon laser trabeculotomy. *Trans Am Acad Ophthalmol Otolaryngol*. 1974;78:371-375.

26. Wise JB, Witter SL. Argon laser therapy for open-angle glaucoma. A pilot study. *Arch Ophthalmol*. 1979;97:319-322.

27. Aslanides IM, Katz LJ. Argon laser trabeculoplasty and peripheral iridectomy. In: Yanoff M, Duker JS, eds. *Ophthalmology*. London; Mosby; 1999:12.26.1-4.

28. Schuman JS. New lasers for treating glaucoma. In: American Academy of Ophthalmology, ed. *A LEO Clinical Update Course on Glaucoma*. San Francisco, Calif: American Academy of Ophthalmology; 2000:23-25.

29. Latina MA, Sibayan SA, Shin DH, Noecker RJ, Marcellino G. Q-switched 532-nm Nd:YAG laser trabeculoplasty (selective laser trabeculoplasty): a multicenter, pilot, clinical study. *Ophthalmology*. 1998;105:2082-2090.

30. Latina MA, Tumbocon JA. Selective laser trabeculoplasty: a new treatment option for open angle glaucoma. *Curr Opin Ophthalmol*. 2002;13:94-96.

31. Damji KF, Shah KC, Rock WJ, Bains HS, Hodge WG. Selective laser trabeculoplasty v argon laser trabeculoplasty: a prospective randomised clinical trial. *Br J Ophthalmolol*. 1999;83:718-722.

32. Shields MB. *Textbook of Glaucoma*. 4th ed. Baltimore, Md: Lippincott, Williams and Wilkins; 1998:504.

8

33. Van Buskirk EM. Trabeculectomy: surgical technique. In: Weinreb RN, Mills RP, eds. *Glaucoma Surgery: Principles and Techniques*. San Francisco: American Academy of Ophthalmology; 1998:28-41.

34. Fellman RL. Trabeculectomy. In: Yanoff M, Duker JS, eds. *Ophthalmology*. London: Mosby; 1999:12.30.1-10.

35. Greenfield DS, Gedde SJ. Glaucoma drainage devices: a mini-review. *Vision & Aging*. 2002;2:18-19.

36. Rosenberg LF, Krupin T. Implants in glaucoma surgery. In: Ritch R, Shields MB, Krupin T, eds. *Glaucomas*. St. Louis, Mo: Mosby-Year Book; 1996:1784-1789.

37. Assaad MH, Baerveldt G, Rockwood EJ. Glaucoma drainage devices: pros and cons. *Curr Opin Ophthalmol*. 1999;10:147-153.

38. Tsai JC, Johnson CC, Dietrich MS. The Ahmed shunt vs the Baerveldt shunt for refractory glaucoma: a single surgeon comparison of outcome. *Ophthalmology*. 2003;110:1814-1821.

39. Samuelson TW. Non-penetrating filtration surgery. In: American Academy of Ophthalmology, ed. *A LEO Clinical Update Course on Glaucoma*. San Francisco, Calif: American Academy of Ophthalmology; 2000:39-43.

40. Orzalesi N, Rossetti L, Invernizzi T, Bottoli A, Autelitano A. Effect of timolol, latanoprost, and dorzolamide on circadian IOP in glaucoma or ocular hypertension. *Invest Ophthalmol Vis Sci*. 2000;41:2566-2573.

41. Liu JH, Kripke DF, Twa MD, et al. Twenty-four hour pattern of intraocular pressure in the aging population. *Invest Ophthalmol Vis Sci*. 1999;40:2912-2917.

42. Asrani S, Zeimer R, Wilensky J, Gieser D, Vitale S, Lindenmuth K. Large diurnal fluctuations in intraocular pressure are an independent risk factor in patients with glaucoma. *J Glaucoma*. 2000;9:134-142.

43. Stewart WC. Maximizing medical therapy for glaucoma. *Rev Ophthalmol*. 2002;9:39-41.

44. Mishima HK, Kiuchi Y, Takamatsu M, Racz P, Bito LZ. Circadian intraocular pressure management with latanoprost: diurnal and nocturnal intraocular pressure reduction and increased uveoscleral outflow. *Surv Ophthalmol.* 1997;41 (suppl 2):S139-S144.

45. Lichter PR, Musch DC, Gillespie BW, et al, for the CIGTS Study Group. Interim clinical outcomes in the Collaborative Initial Glaucoma Treatment Study comparing initial treatment randomized to medication or surgery. *Ophthalmology.* 2001;108:1943-1953.

46. Musch DC, Lichter PR, Guire KE, Standardi CL. The Collaborative Initial Glaucoma Treatment Study: study design, methods, and baseline characteristics. *Ophthalmology.* 1999;106:653-662.

47. Kriegelstein GK. Medical treatment of glaucoma. In: Hitchings RA, ed. *Glaucoma.* London: BMJ Publishing Group; 2000:77-84.

48. Tsai JC, McClure CA, Ramos SE, Schlundt DG, Pichert JW. Compliance barriers in glaucoma: a systemic classification. *J Glaucoma.* 2003;12:393-398.

49. Claxton AJ, Cramer J, Pierce C. A systematic review of the associations between dose regimens and medication compliance. *Clin Ther.* 2001;23:1296-1310.

50. Patel SC, Spaeth GL. Compliance in patients prescribed eyedrops for glaucoma. *Ophthalmic Surg.* 1995;26:233-236.

51. Kass MA, Meltzer DW, Gordon M, Cooper D, Goldberg J. Compliance with topical pilocarpine treatment. *Am J Ophthalmol.* 1986;101:515-523.

52. Goldberg I. Compliance. In: Ritch R, Shields MB, Krupin T, eds. *Glaucomas.* 2nd ed. St. Louis, Mo: Mosby-Year Book; 1996:1375-1384.

53. Kobelt G, Jonsson L, Gerdtham U, Krieglstein G. Direct costs of glaucoma management following initiation of medical therapy. A simulation model based on an observational study of glaucoma treatment in Germany. *Graefes Arch Clin Exp Ophthalmol.* 1998;236:811-823.

8

54. American Academy of Ophthalmology Preferred Practice Patterns Committee Glaucoma Panel. *Preferred Practice Patterns. Primary Open-Angle Glaucoma.* San Francisco, Calif: American Academy of Ophthalmology; 2000:1-38.

55. Fechtner RD, Singh K. Maximal glaucoma therapy. *J Glaucoma.* 2001;10(5 suppl 1):S73-S75.

56. Weinreb RN. Lowering intraocular pressure to minimize glaucoma damage. *J Glaucoma.* 2001;10(5 suppl 1):S76-S77.

57. Leske MC, Heijl A, Hussein M, Bengtsson B, Hyman L, Komaroff E; Early Manifest Glaucoma Trial Group. Factors for glaucoma progression and the effect of treatment: the early manifest glaucoma trial. *Arch Ophthalmol.* 2003; 121:48-56.

58. Ritch R, Shields MB, Krupin T. Chronic open-angle glaucoma treatment. In: Ritch R, Shields MB, Krupin T, eds. *Glaucomas.* 2nd ed. St. Louis, Mo: Mosby-Year Book; 1996:1507-1519.

59. Smith J, Wandel T. Rationale for the one-eye therapeutic trial. *Ann Ophthalmol.* 1986;18:8.

60. Zimmerman TJ, Kooner KS, Kandarakis AS, Ziegler LP. Improving the therapeutic index of topically applied ocular drugs. *Arch Ophthalmol.* 1984;102:551-553.

61. Huang TC, Lee DA. Punctal occlusion and topical medications for glaucoma. *Am J Ophthalmol.* 1989;107:151-155.

9 Landmark Glaucoma Studies

A number of pivotal clinical studies have established the role of elevated intraocular pressure (IOP) in the progression of glaucoma and the efficacy of different therapeutic strategies (medication, laser surgery, or filtering surgery) in controlling IOP and preventing disease progression. These studies have been instrumental in providing guidelines that assist in the establishment of algorithms for management of glaucoma (**Table 9.1**).

Glaucoma Laser Trial

The Glaucoma Laser Trial (GLT) compared the efficacy and safety of argon laser trabeculoplasty (ALT) as an alternative to topical ocular hypotensive medications as initial therapy in controlling IOP in patients with primary open-angle glaucoma (POAG).[1] In this multicenter trial, 271 patients with newly diagnosed, previously untreated POAG had one eye randomly assigned to receive timolol maleate (0.5%) as primary therapy and ALT in the other eye. A stepped regimen for additional medication was administered for uncontrolled IOP in either eye.

During the 2-year follow-up, the ALT eyes had lower mean IOPs (1-2 mm Hg) than medically treated eyes, and fewer ALT eyes required simultaneous prescription of two or more medications. In addition, at the end of 2 years, 44% of eyes were controlled by ALT alone, 70% were controlled by ALT or ALT and timolol, and 89% were controlled with the stepped medication regimen (ie, other medications added to ALT and timolol). In contrast, 30% of eyes treated with

TABLE 9.1 — SUMMARY OF LANDMARK GLAUCOMA STUDIES

Study	Objective	Implications
Glaucoma Laser Trial (GLT)	To determine efficacy and safety of ALT as an alternative to topical medication for controlling IOP in glaucoma	After 2 years of follow-up, more eyes were controlled by initial treatment with ALT than by initial treatment with timolol. There were no significant differences between the two groups with regard to visual acuity or VF. Thus, ALT may be an alternative to medication as initial treatment for glaucoma. (Note: Study was completed prior to introduction of prostaglandin analogues, topical CAIs, and α-agonists)
Collaborative Normal-Tension Glaucoma Study (CNTGS)	To determine if IOP is involved in the pathogenesis of NTG	IOP is indeed part of pathogenic process in NTG. Therapy that is effective in lowering IOP and is free of adverse effects may be beneficial for patients with NTG. However, a 30% reduction of IOP was required in this study, an aggressive goal that may require therapeutic regimens that cause adverse ocular effects. Since 65% of untreated eyes showed no progression, the decision to treat aggressively must be weighed against the individual likelihood of progression

Advanced Glaucoma Intervention Study (AGIS)	To compare the outcome of ALT first vs trabeculectomy first as intervention for advanced glaucoma refractory to medical therapy. Also to determine relationship between IOP level and VF deterioration	Low IOP is associated with reduced progression of VF deterioration and optic neuropathy. Patients with IOP maintained <18 mm Hg for length of study (average 12.3 mm Hg, over 6 years) had near zero VF loss. This study suggests aggressive medical management for baseline IOP values >17.5 mm Hg
Collaborative Initial Glaucoma Treatment Study (CIGTS)	To compare the efficacy of initial glaucoma treatment with medication or trabeculectomy surgery	VF loss was similar in both treatment groups, the rate of cataract removal was higher in the surgery group, average IOP was slightly lower with surgery, and visual acuity loss was greater with surgery in the short-term but similar after 4 years of treatment. The study indicated that medical treatment provides benefits comparable to those of trabeculectomy surgery in the initial treatment of glaucoma. These results do not warrant changing the currently recommended medication first treatment approach

Continued

9

Study	Objective	Implications
Early Manifest Glaucoma Trial (EMGT)	To compare the effect of immediate lowering of IOP vs no treatment on the progression of newly detected OAG	After a median follow-up of 6 years, progression was less frequent in the treatment group (45%) than in the control no treatment group (62%) and occurred significantly later in treated patients
The Ocular Hypertension Treatment Study (OHTS)	To determine the efficacy of topical ocular hypotensive medications in preventing or delaying the onset of POAG in patients with ocular hypertension	There was significantly less cumulative probability of developing POAG in the treated eyes compared with the control eyes and little evidence of ocular risk associated with medication. This study demonstrated that topical ocular hypotensives are effective in reducing the incidence of glaucomatous field loss in individuals with elevated IOP. These results were achieved with a moderate (only 20%) reduction in IOP from baseline that was maintained over 72 months of follow-up.

| Central Corneal Thickness in the OHTS | The study determined that CCT does influence the measurement of IOP and that IOP in patients with thicker corneas will be overestimated (conversely, IOP in patients with thinner corneas will be underestimated). Thus CCT may influence the accuracy of applanation tonometry with regard to the diagnosis, screening, and management of patients with glaucoma and ocular hypertension. Furthermore, corneal thickness should be accounted for in any risk model for glaucoma |

Abbreviations: ALT, argon laser trabeculoplasty; CAI, carbonic anhydrase inhibitor; CCT, central corneal thickness; IOP, intraocular pressure; NTG, normal-tension glaucoma; OAG, open-angle glaucoma; POAG, primary open-angle glaucoma; VF, visual field.

9

117

timolol remained controlled on this regimen, with 66% controlled by stepped medication. Visual acuity and visual field showed no significant differences between the groups. At the 7- to 9-year follow-up, eyes treated initially with ALT had a 1.2 mm Hg greater reduction in IOP (P <0.001) and 0.6 dB lower perimetric mean deviation (P <0.001) compared with eyes treated initially with medication. There was no significant difference in the change in cup-disc (C/D) ratio.

The results of this study suggest that trabeculoplasty may be considered as first-line therapy for patients newly diagnosed with POAG (especially patients intolerant of medical therapy). It is important to note, however, that the GLT was performed prior to the introduction of the PG analogues (eg, latanoprost), topical carbonic anhydrase inhibitors (eg, dorzolamide), and α_2-agonists (eg, brimonidine).

The Collaborative Normal-Tension Glaucoma Study

The Collaborative Normal-Tension Glaucoma Study (CNTGS) sought to determine whether IOP is a factor in the pathogenesis of normal-tension glaucoma (NTG).[2] One eye of each patient was randomized to receive either no treatment or to have sufficient treatment consisting of medications, laser, and/or incisional surgery to lower IOP by 30% from baseline. Eyes were eligible if they met the criteria for NTG and showed progression or high-risk visual field defects. Of 140 eyes (140 patients), 79 (56%) were randomized to no treatment and 61 (44%) were randomized to treatment.

There was a statistically significant favorable effect of lowering IOP by 30% on visual field and optic disk deterioration (P <0.001) compared with the untreated group. The study investigators concluded that IOP is indeed involved in the pathology of NTG, that therapy is effective in lowering IOP, and that, free of adverse effects, IOP reduction of a 30% magnitude is beneficial in patients who are at risk of their disease progressing. However, because 65% of untreated patients showed no progression during follow-up, the natural history of NTG must be considered in the choice of therapy to lower IOP (with various side effects of therapy including exacerbation of cataract formation due to surgery in the treated group), unless NTG poses a serious threat of visual loss.[3]

Advanced Glaucoma Intervention Study

The Advanced Glaucoma Intervention Study (AGIS) involved randomization of 789 eyes (of 591 patients) with advanced open-angle glaucoma (OAG) refractory to medical therapy to compare the long-term outcome of two sequences of intervention. The sequences to be compared were ALT first, to be followed (as needed) by trabeculectomy and then repeat trabeculectomy (ATT), vs trabeculectomy first, to be followed (as needed) by ALT and then repeat trabeculectomy (TAT). Patients were examined every 6 months following enrollment, the initial intervention, and an initial series of visits. After 7 years of follow-up, the mean decrease in IOP was greater in eyes that underwent trabeculectomy first (TAT), and the rate of failure following initial intervention was greater for eyes treated with ALT first (ATT).[4] In white patients, the better IOP control achieved by the trabeculectomy first sequence resulted in better visual outcomes, both visual field and visual acuity. In black patients, however, the visual outcomes (both visual field and visual acuity) were better for eyes treated with ALT first despite better IOP control for eyes treated with trabeculectomy first.[5]

In addition to the original objective, the extensive AGIS data were also used to analyze the relationship between IOP levels and visual field deterioration. A predictive analysis[6] was done to determine whether

IOP values during the early follow-up period are predictive of subsequent changes from baseline in visual field defect scores. Patients were grouped into three categories based on IOP ranges over the first 18 months: <14 mm Hg, 14 to 17.5 mg Hg, and >17.5 mm Hg. The mean change (from baseline) in visual field defect scores at each 6-month period was calculated for each specific range of IOP values (**Figure 9**.1).

A second associative analysis[6] determined the percentage of visits over the first 6 years of follow-up for which the measured IOP was <18 mm Hg. There were four categories in this analysis: 100% of all visits, 75% to <100%, 50% to <75%, and 0% to <50%. Here, too, the mean change (from baseline) of visual field defect scores at each 6-month period was calculated for each category.

Both the predictive and associative analyses demonstrated that dramatic lowering of IOP is associated with reduced progression of visual field defects. Initial IOP values >17.5 mm Hg resulted in worsening of visual defect scores of one unit over an initial follow-up period of 18 months. Eyes that experienced the lowest IOP—those maintaining IOP <18 mm Hg 100% of the time over the 6-year follow-up period (with an average IOP of 12.3 mm Hg)—had a near zero change in visual defect scores. In this maximum IOP-controlled group, there was an improvement in visual field scores during the first 2 years (–0.26) and minor worsening after 4 years (0.46). Overall, the AGIS results provide strong support for previous expert opinions that achieving low levels of IOP slows progression of visual deterioration.

Collaborative Initial Glaucoma Treatment Study

The Collaborative Initial Glaucoma Treatment Study (CIGTS) randomized 607 patients with newly-diagnosed OAG, selecting one eye from each patient,

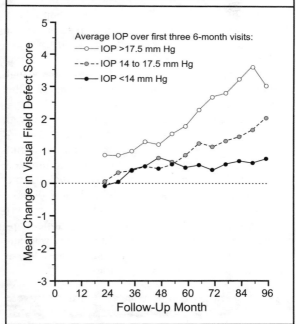

FIGURE 9.1 — AGIS PREDICTIVE ANALYSIS: MEAN CHANGE FROM BASELINE IN VISUAL FIELD DEFECT SCORE

Average IOP over first three 6-month visits:
- ·····○····· IOP >17.5 mm Hg
- --●-- IOP 14 to 17.5 mm Hg
- ——●—— IOP <14 mm Hg

Mean Change in Visual Field Defect Score

Follow-Up Month

Abbreviation: IOP, intraocular pressure.

The AGIS Investigators: The Advanced Glaucoma Intervention Study (AGIS) 7. *Am J Ophthalmol.* 2000;130:429-440.

to be treated with either medication first or filtering surgery (trabeculectomy) first.[7] Patients were treated aggressively to lower IOP to a predetermined target level and were evaluated every 6 months over 5 years. Primary outcome was visual field loss with visual acuity being a secondary outcome of the study.

Visual field loss did not differ significantly between the two groups after 5 years, although the surgically treated patients had an initial increased risk of substantial visual acuity loss compared with the medically treated patients. After 4 years follow-up, the average visual acuities in the two groups were the same. The surgical group averaged a lower IOP (14 to 15 mm Hg) compared with the medication group (17 to 18 mm Hg), but the former group of patients had a greater rate of cataract removal. In conclusion, the CIGTS demonstrated that both initial medication and initial surgical treatment produced comparable visual field outcomes after 5 years of follow-up and that the difference in visual acuities converged over that time.

The CIGTS suggests that the benefits derived from medication therapy are comparable to those derived from trabeculectomy; aggressive and successful IOP lowering by either treatment modality minimized visual field loss. The investigators concluded that the results from their 5-year study (of a chronic disease such as glaucoma) do not warrant changing the currently recommended medication "first" treatment approach. The initial posttreatment visual acuity was better in the medication first group because of the adverse impact of filtration surgery on vision.

Early Manifest Glaucoma Trial

The Early Manifest Glaucoma Trial (EMGT) was a prospective, randomized clinical trial that compared the effect of immediate lowering of IOP vs no treatment or later treatment on the progression of newly detected OAG.[8] Patients were randomized to either laser trabeculoplasty plus topical betaxolol treatment or no initial treatment. A significant number of them had a diagnosis of NTG.

On average, treatment lowered IOP by approximately 5 mm Hg (or 25% from a median baseline IOP of 20 mm Hg). Progression was seen less frequently in treated patients (45%) than in untreated control patients (62%) and occurred significantly later in the former group. The beneficial effects of treatment were

122

present in both older and younger patients, in high- and normal-tension glaucoma, and in eyes with less and greater visual field loss.

Ocular Hypertension Study

The Ocular Hypertension Study (OHTS) was a large, long-term, multicenter randomized trial to determine whether topical ocular hypotensive medications are effective in delaying or preventing the onset of POAG in subjects without evidence of glaucomatous damage. The safety of these IOP-lowering medications was evaluated as well.[9] A total of 1636 subjects with an IOP between 24 mm Hg and 32 mm Hg in one eye and between 21 mm Hg and 32 mm Hg in the other eye were randomized to receive either treatment with all types of commercially available topical ocular hypotensives (817 patients) or observation without treatment (819 patients). The goal in the medication group was to reduce IOP by 20% or more from baseline and to achieve an IOP of ≤24 mm Hg.

The primary outcome was the development of a reproducible visual field abnormality or reproducible optic disc deterioration attributable to POAG in one or both eyes. The mean reduction of IOP in the medication group was 22.5% compared with 4.0% in the observation group. After 60 months, the cumulative probability of developing POAG was 4.4% in the medication group vs 9.5% in the observation group, a statistically significant difference (P <0.0001). There was also a treatment benefit observed for reproducible visual field abnormality attributed to POAG (P = 0.002) and for reproducible optic disc deterioration (P <0.001).

There was no evidence of excess risk in the medication group for participant-reported symptoms or for overall number of new medical conditions, worsening of preexisting conditions, hospitalizations, or mortality. However, it was noted that ocular hypotensive medications might cause more adverse effects in routine practice than occurred in this clinical trial. The OHTS clearly demonstrated that topical ocular hypotensive medication(s) was effective in delaying or preventing the onset of POAG in individuals with elevated IOP. It also demonstrated that moderate IOP reductions could be achieved and maintained during a 72-month follow-up period.

In an accompanying article,[10] proportional hazards models were used to identify baseline factors that predicted the development of POAG in the OHTS. Based on multivariate analyses, baseline age, vertical and horizontal C/D ratio, pattern standard deviation, and IOP were all noted to be good predictors for the onset of POAG. In addition, subjects with thinner central corneal measurements were at greater risk for developing POAG (see below).

Corneal Thickness and Intraocular Pressure Measurement

In another phase of the OHTS, Brandt and associates[11] analyzed the data from central corneal thickness (CCT) measurements by ultrasonic pachymetry on 1301 of the 1636 subjects. Compared with a normal value of 544 microns, the mean values were 573 microns for the entire group, 579 microns for the 912 Caucasians, and 556 microns for the 318 African Americans. Of special interest, 24% of the group measured >600 microns.

In a subsequent OHTS report,[10] CCT was found to be a powerful predictor for development of POAG, even after adjusting for the effects of IOP, age, C/D ratio, and perimetric pattern standard deviation. The risk of developing POAG was inversely correlated with CCT. Participants with CCT ≤555 microns had a threefold greater risk than those with CCT >588 microns. These findings are consistent with prior knowledge that corneal thickness influences measurement of IOP by

Goldmann tonometry such that true IOP is overestimated in eyes with thicker corneas and underestimated in eyes with thinner corneas. It has become evident that CCT is an essential parameter for monitoring patients with ocular hypertension (some may have nothing more than thick corneas) and for treating patients with glaucoma.

Summary

The OHTS investigators cautioned that their study results do not suggest that all individuals with elevated IOP should be treated with topical ocular hypotensive medication. The decision to initiate therapy in patients with elevated IOP but without signs of glaucomatous damage should be based on the individual's risk for POAG, health status, and life expectancy. The burdens of long-term treatment and the potential for adverse effects must be factored into the decision, as well as the fact that population-based studies have demonstrated that there is a low overall incidence of POAG in individuals with OH. The OHTS results, taken together with the CNTGS, CITGS, EMGT, and AGIS results, provide strong evidence that lowering IOP is protective in all varieties of OAG.

9

REFERENCES

1. The Glaucoma Laser Trial Research Group. The Glaucoma Laser Trial (GLT). 2. Results of argon laser trabeculoplasty versus topical medications. *Ophthalmology.* 1990;97:1403-1413.

2. Collaborative Normal-Tension Glaucoma Study Group. The effectiveness of intraocular pressure reduction in the treatment of normal-tension glaucoma. *Am J Ophthalmol.* 1998; 126:498-505.

3. Collaborative Normal-Tension Glaucoma Study Group. Comparison of glaucomatous progression between untreated patients with normal-tension glaucoma and patients with therapeutically reduced intraocular pressures. *Am J Ophthalmol.* 1998;126:487-497.

4. The Advanced Glaucoma Intervention Study (AGIS): 4. Comparison of treatment outcomes within race. Seven-year results. *Ophthalmology*. 1998;105:1146-1164.

5. The Advanced Glaucoma Intervention Study (AGIS): 9. Comparison of glaucoma outcomes in black and white patients within treatment groups. *Am J Ophthalmol*. 2001;132:311-320.

6. The Advanced Glaucoma Intervention Study (AGIS): 7. The relationship between control of intraocular pressure and visual field deterioration. The AGIS Investigators. *Am J Ophthalmol*. 2000;130:429-440.

7. Lichter PR, Musch DC, Gillespie BW, et al, for the CIGTS Study Group. Interim clinical outcomes in the Collaborative Initial Glaucoma Treatment Study comparing initial treatment randomized to medication or surgery. *Ophthalmology*. 2001;108:1943-1953.

8. Heijl A, Leske MC, Bengtsson B, et al. Reduction of intraocular pressure and glaucoma progression. Results from the Early Manifest Glaucoma Trial. *Arch Ophthalmol*. 2002; 120:1268-1279.

9. Kass MA, Heuer DK, Higginbotham EJ, et al. The Ocular Hypertension Treatment Study: a randomized trial determines that topical ocular hypotensive medication delays or prevents the onset of primary open-angle glaucoma. *Arch Ophthalmol*. 2002;120:701-713.

10. Gordon MO, Beiser JA, Brandt JD, et al. The Ocular Hypertension Treatment Study: baseline factors that predict the onset of primary open-angle glaucoma. *Arch Ophthalmol*. 2002;120:714-720.

11. Brandt JD, Beiser JA, Kass MA, Gordon MO. Central corneal thickness in the Ocular Hypertension Treatment Study (OHTS). *Ophthalmology*. 2001;108:1779-1788.

10 Medications for Glaucoma

Medications that control intraocular pressure (IOP), both oral and topical ocular hypotensives, exert their action by:

- Inhibiting aqueous humor production (**Table 8.2**)
- Enhancing aqueous outflow (**Table 8.3**)
- Or doing both.

β-Antagonists

β-Blockers have been a mainstay of topical ocular hypotensive therapy. They include both noncardioselective and cardioselective (β_1-adrenergic) receptor blockers.[1] Characteristics of currently available β-blockers are shown in **Table 10.1**.

■ Efficacy

The topical β-blockers are indicated for the treatment of elevated IOP in patients with open-angle glaucoma (OAG) or ocular hypertension (OH).[2] Timolol was the first topical β-blocker used as an ocular hypotensive for glaucoma in the United States and is considered the gold standard against which all other topical agents are compared. It is effective in significantly lowering IOP and protecting against glaucomatous field loss and glaucomatous optic neuropathy (GON). As a class, the other topical β-blockers display efficacy similar to that of timolol, although betaxolol has been shown to be less effective in lowering IOP.[3] In addition, Schuman reported that timolol-treated patients concurrently taking systemic β-blocker therapy had decreased efficacy (ie, smaller decreases in IOP) and greater systemic side effects (ie, greater changes in systolic and diastolic blood pressures and

TABLE 10.1 — β-ADRENERGIC ANTAGONISTS USED AS OCULAR HYPOTENSIVES FOR GLAUCOMA			
Generic (Trade) Name	**Concentration (%)**	**Cardioselectivity**	**Dosage**
Betaxolol (Betoptic)	0.5	+	1 drop bid
Betaxolol (Betoptic S)	0.25	+	1 drop bid
Carteolol (Ocupress)	1.0	–	1 drop bid
Levobunolol (Betagan)	0.25, 0.5	–	1 drop bid
Metipranolol (OptiPranol)	0.3	–	1 drop bid
Timolol hemihydrate (Betimol)	0.25, 0.5	–	1 drop bid
Timolol maleate (Timoptic)	0.25, 0.5	–	1 drop bid
Timolol maleate gel (Timoptic-XE)	0.25 gel, 0.5 gel	–	1 drop qd

greater decreases in heart rate) when compared with timolol-treated subjects not taking systemic β-blocker medication.[4]

■ Ocular Side Effects

Although ocular side effects (such as stinging, burning, redness, blurred vision, and foreign-body sensation) are associated with topical β-blockers, their occurrence is low and diminishes with time. However, one notable adverse event associated with metipranolol is granulomatous uveitis.[5,6]

■ Systemic Side Effects

A greater concern with the topical β-blockers is the potential for systemic side effects, which are similar to those associated with systemic β-blockers (**Table 10.2**). It is important to note that betaxolol, a cardioselective β-blocker, has less potential for causing the pulmonary adverse events associated with nonselective β-blockers. Though betaxolol may be the β-blocker of choice in patients with asthma or other bronchospastic pulmonary disorders, it should be dispensed with caution and careful monitoring in these patients.[7] Given the extent and severity of serious systemic adverse effects that can occur with topical β-blocker therapy, alternative and better-tolerated agents that are equally or more effective in controlling IOP may be appropriate when starting glaucoma therapy.[5]

■ Contraindications

In addition to hypersensitivity to any of the components of a particular agent, the range of contraindications, which apply to most topical β-blockers, include:

- Sinus bradycardia
- Second- or third-degree heart block
- Cardiogenic shock
- Overt cardiac failure

TABLE 10.2 — TYPICAL SYSTEMIC ADVERSE EFFECTS OF TOPICAL β-BLOCKERS
Cardiovascular   • Arrhythmia   • Bradycardia   • Cardiac arrest   • Cardiac failure   • Heart block   • Hypertension   • Hypotension   • Syncope
Respiratory   • Bronchospasm*   • Cough   • Dyspnea   • Respiratory failure
Nervous system   • Confusion   • Depression   • Dizziness   • Headache   • Insomnia   • Nightmares   • Somnolence
* Predominantly in individuals with pre-existing respiratory failure.

- Bronchial asthma
- Severe chronic obstructive pulmonary disease.

■ Drug Interactions

The systemic absorption of topical β-blockers can have profound cardiovascular effects. Therefore, β-blockers should be prescribed with caution in patients with comorbidities that require taking drugs that affect the cardiovascular system because there is enhanced potential for serious additive adverse effects. This is particularly relevant for patients who are already taking systemic β-blockers. Drug reactions can also occur when topical β-blockers are prescribed in patients taking adrenergic psychotropic drugs, catecholamine-depleting drugs, calcium antagonists, or digitalis.[3]

Prostaglandin Analogues

■ **Efficacy**

Prostaglandin (PG) analogues are among the newest topical ocular hypotensive medications for glaucoma and have been available since the release of latanoprost in 1996.[8] Since that time, three other PG derivatives have become available for the topical treatment of glaucoma, and all produce significant and sustained lowering of IOP (**Table 10.3**). As will be seen in Chapter 11, *Comparative Clinical Trials/Primary Treatment Algorithm*, clinical studies have shown that all PG analogues, with the exception of unoprostone, reduce IOP to a significantly greater degree than timolol.[9-14]

In December 2002, latanoprost (Xalatan) received a first-line use for the treatment of OAG or OH from the United States Food and Drug Administration (FDA). Latanoprost also has a first-line indication in Japan and throughout Europe. In contrast, the other three PG analogues (bimatoprost, travoprost, and unoprostone) are indicated for the treatment of OAG or OH in patients who are intolerant of other IOP-lowering medications or fail to achieve a target response with these other medications.[3] Pending further developments, they are still to be prescribed as second-line therapy.

PG analogues offer significant advantages over β-blockers.[15] PG analogues:
- Are more effective in lowering IOP than β-blockers over the diurnal cycle (both day and night)
- Increase outflow rather than suppress aqueous production

TABLE 10.3 — PROSTAGLANDIN ANALOGUES USED IN THE TREATMENT OF GLAUCOMA

Generic (Trade) Name	Concentration (%)	IOP Reduction (mm Hg) (% reduction)	Dosage
Latanoprost (Xalatan)	0.005	6-8 (24-32)	1 drop qhs
Bimatoprost (Lumigan)	0.03	7-8 (27-31)	1 drop qhs
Travoprost (Travatan)	0.004	6-8 (23-32)	1 drop qhs
Unoprostone (Rescula)	0.15	3-4 (13-17)	1 drop bid

Abbreviation: IOP, intraocular pressure.

Physicians' Desk Reference for Ophthalmic Medicines: 2004. Montvale, NJ: Thomson Healthcare; 2003.

- Are about 100 times more potent than topical β-blockers
- Possess a safer systemic side-effect profile
- Have a simpler dosing schedule (except for unoprostone).

Due to their marked efficacy in controlling 24-hour IOP, the low incidence of systemic side effects, and the other advantages listed above, there has been a recent paradigm shift toward considering PG analogues (rather than β-blockers) as first-line therapy for initial control of IOP in patients with glaucoma. In addition, a recent study demonstrated that latanoprost produces a greater rate of IOP response than timolol in patients with OH or glaucoma (several criteria were used to define a "responder" including a specified percentage reduction of IOP, a specified change in IOP in mm Hg, or a specified final absolute IOP achieved).[16]

■ Contraindications

Contraindications for all of the PG analogues include sensitivity to the particular agent, the benzalkonium chloride preservative, or any other ingredient in the product. In addition, relative contraindications for use of PG analogues occur in patients with active iridocyclitis and/or known history of herpes simplex keratitis and history of cystoid macular edema (CME).

■ Warnings

All of the PG analogues have been reported to cause changes in ocular pigment tissues that may be permanent. For latanoprost, travoprost, and bimatoprost, these changes include:
- Increased pigmentation of the iris and periorbital tissue (eyelid)
- Increased pigmentation and growth of eyelashes.

■ **Side Effects**

Since the concentration of any PG analogue entering the systemic circulation is considerably lower than that of circulating endogenous PGs, there have been few reports of significant systemic toxicity. Nevertheless, there are a number of ocular side effects that warrant consideration. **Table 10.4** reviews the systemic and ocular side effects associated with the PG analogues.

There is a high occurrence of conjunctival hyperemia for travoprost (35% to 50%) and bimatoprost (15% to 45%). Approximately 3% of patients discontinue therapy with each of these agents. In contrast, only 5% to 15% of patients on latanoprost experience conjunctival hyperemia and <1% of these patients discontinue therapy due to this specific side effect.

■ **Cystoid Macular Edema and Latanoprost**

Although CME has been reported with the use of latanoprost and other PG analogues, the number of involved eyes has been relatively few when compared with the number of eyes that have been treated with these agents. Altogether, there have been 32 published cases (and <150 reported cases) of CME during latanoprost treatment in the 3 years following its introduction in 1996[17,18] (out of an estimated 3.3 million patients treated with this PG analogue).[19] Furthermore, a number of studies that have investigated the association between latanoprost therapy and CME have failed to establish a direct cause-and-effect relationship.[17,18,20-22] Of note is that in almost all of the published reports of latanoprost-induced CME, patients had a number of other established risk factors for CME, including:
- Torn posterior capsule
- Prior uveitis
- Prior cataract surgery (with resultant aphakia or pseudophakia)

- Ocular inflammation
- Complicated surgery.[18]

In addition, when latanoprost was discontinued in these cases, the CME resolved.[17,18] Hence, PG analogues should be used with caution in eyes that are prone to CME.

α-Agonists

There are currently two selective α_2-agonists used to lower IOP (**Table 10.5**):
- Apraclonidine hydrochloride
- Brimonidine tartrate.

■ Indications

Apraclonidine (0.5%) is indicated in most cases for short-term adjunctive use in patients already on maximum tolerable medical therapy who require additional IOP reduction. Treatment should be discontinued if IOP rises significantly. Apraclonidine (1.0%) is indicated to control or prevent the postsurgical increases in IOP associated with laser surgery.

Brimonidine is used in the majority of cases when an α_2-agonist is needed for long-term, sustained therapy. Both formulations of brimonidine (0.15% and 0.2%) are indicated for the lowering of IOP in patients with OAG or OH.[3] At this time, brimonidine (0.15%) (Alphagan P) is the only formulation of the drug commercially available. This lower dose formulation with purite preservative has a reduced incidence of allergic conjunctivitis, better satisfaction and comfort rating, and similar IOP lowering when compared with the standard 0.2% concentration.[23]

■ Efficacy

When an α_2-agonist is added to a regimen of two aqueous-suppressing agents, such as a β-blocker plus

10

TABLE 10.4 — OCULAR AND SYSTEMIC SIDE EFFECTS OF PROSTAGLANDIN ANALOGUES USED TO TREAT GLAUCOMA

Adverse Event	Occurrence (%)			
	Latanoprost	Travoprost	Bimatoprost	Unoprostone
Ocular				
Blurred vision	5-15	1-4	3-10	5-10
Burning and/or stinging	5-15	—	3-10	10-25
Cataract	—	1-4	3-10	1-5
Conjunctivitis	<1	1-4	1-3	1-5
Cystoid macula edema	*	*	*	*
Dry eye	1-4	1-4	3-10	10-25
Eyelid skin darkening	*	*	3-10	<1
Eyelash growth/changes	*	*	15-45	10-25
Foreign-body sensation	5-15	5-10	3-10	5-10

Hyperemia	5-15	35-50	15-45	10-25
Iris discoloration	5-15	1-4	1-3	<1
Pain	1-4	5-10	3-10	1-5
Iritis	*	*	<1	<1
Systemic				
Allergic reaction	1-2	—	—	1-5
Chest pain/angina pectoris	1-2	1-5	—	—
Headache	—	1-5	1-5	1-5
Muscle, joint, or back pain	1-2	1-5	—	1-5
Upper respiratory infection (ie, flu-like symptoms)	4	1-5	10	6

* Postmarketing case reports.

Physicians' Desk Reference for Ophthalmic Medicines: 2004. Montvale, NJ: Thomson Healthcare; 2003.

10

TABLE 10.5 — α_2-AGONISTS USED IN THE TREATMENT OF GLAUCOMA			
Generic (Trade) Name	Concentration (%)	IOP Reduction (mm Hg)	Dosage
Apraclonidine hydrochloride (Iopidine)	0.5	5-6	1 drop tid (bid also used)
Apraclonidine hydrochloride (Iopidine)	1.0	NA	1 drop pre- and 1 drop postoperatively (laser)
Brimonidine tartrate (Alphagan P)	0.15	2-5	1 drop tid (bid often used)
Briminodine tartrate (Alphagan)	0.2	4-6	1 drop tid (bid often used)

Abreviation: IOP, intraocular pressure; NA, not available.

Data for IOP reduction with apraclonidine 0.5% adapted from: Nagasubramanian S, et al. *Ophthalmology.* 1993;100:1318; and data also from: *Physicians' Desk Reference for Ophthalmic Medicines: 2004.* Montvale, NJ: Thomson Healthcare; 2003.

a carbonic anhydrase inhibitor (CAI), there may be minimal additional IOP lowering, since a third aqueous suppressant may not add much IOP effect. Tachyphylaxis is common with apraclonidine, and its benefit may be limited to a duration of 1 month. The efficacy of brimonidine (0.2%) may also diminish with time in some patients.

In clinical studies, apraclonidine (1%) successfully controlled or prevented the postsurgical IOP rise commonly seen following laser surgery. In the placebo-treated eyes, IOP spikes ranged from 2.5 to 8.4 mm Hg. The difference between the two groups was significant (P <0.05). Apraclonidine (0.5%) was also demonstrated to successfully control IOP and delay surgery (when compared with placebo) in patients on maximum tolerated medical therapy.[3] In another trial, apraclonidine (0.5%) was shown to be as effective as timolol in lowering IOP over a 90-day period.[24]

In comparative clinical studies, brimonidine (0.2%) was shown to be comparable to timolol (0.5%) in lowering IOP in patients with glaucoma (4 to 6 mm Hg for brimonidine vs 6 mm Hg for timolol). In other clinical studies, brimonidine (0.15%) was found to be comparable in efficacy to brimonidine (0.2%).[3,23]

■ **Contraindications**

Both apraclonidine and brimonidine are contraindicated in patients hypersensitive to either product or any component of the medications, and in patients receiving monoamine oxidase (MAO) inhibitors. Apraclonidine is also contraindicated in patients who are hypersensitive to clonidine. With brimonidine in particular, caution should be exercised in patients susceptible to side effects of fatigue, drowsiness, somnolence, and dry mouth. Brimonidine should not be used in infants and young children due to increased risks of lethargy and somnolence.

■ **Drug Interactions**

Apraclonidine should not be used with MAO inhibitors, and there may be some potentiating or additive effects with central nervous system depressants. In addition, caution should be used in coadministering apraclonidine with β-blockers since the resultant combination may increase the risk of cardiovascular side effects (eg, reduced blood pressure and heart rate). With regard to brimonidine, the same precautions as for apraclonidine may be prudent.

■ **Side Effects**

Adverse events that occur with apraclonidine and brimonidine are listed in **Table 10.6**. Since brimonidine is often used for long-term, sustained therapy as compared with the shorter-term use of apraclonidine, careful attention should be directed toward the late onset development of ocular and systemic side effects with the former. When used as monotherapy, apraclonidine has minimal cardiovascular effects and does not significantly affect either the heart rate or blood pressure. In contrast, brimonidine may produce some degree of hypotension with long-term use. In addition, some patients may develop allergic follicular conjunctivitis that may require discontinuing this agent. In general, brimonidine has demonstrated a favorable side-effect profile with few discontinuations of therapy.[2,5]

Topical Carbonic Anhydrase Inhibitors

There are currently two topical CAIs indicated for the treatment of elevated IOP in patients with OAG and ocular hypotension (**Table 10.7**):
- Dorzolamide hydrochloride (2%)
- Brinzolamide (1%).

■ **Efficacy**

Topical CAIs were introduced as an alternative to oral CAIs, which are associated with a wide range of serious side effects (discussed below). Topical CAIs have been shown to reduce IOP by up to 24% as monotherapy and provide an additional 15% reduction when added to timolol.[5] In a yearlong trial comparing dorzolamide with timolol (0.5%) and betaxolol (0.5%), dorzolamide was found to have an IOP-lowering effect similar to the other two—23% compared with 25% for timolol and 21% for betaxolol.[25]

■ **Contraindications, Warnings, and Drug Interactions**

Known contraindications to use of the topical CAIs include hypersensitivity to either of the agents and any component of the products. Since topical CAIs are absorbed systemically, similar adverse reactions to those seen with the oral forms may occur, although with much less frequency. If any such reactions occur, topical CAI therapy should be discontinued.[3] Although no specific drug interactions have been demonstrated with the topical CAIs, they have occurred with the oral CAI agents; specifically, when taken with salicylates.

■ **Adverse Events**

Adverse reactions that occur with topical CAIs are provided in **Table 10.8**.[3] Although the systemic side effects of topical CAIs have been shown to be considerably less than for oral agents, there is still the potential for serious side effects due to systemic absorption of these agents. More clinical studies are needed to evaluate their systemic effects. Significant ocular side effects, such as corneal decompensation and hypotony, have also been reported with the topical CAI agents.[5]

TABLE 10.6 — OCULAR AND SYSTEMIC SIDE EFFECTS OF α₂-AGONISTS USED IN THE TREATMENT OF GLAUCOMA

Side Effect	Occurrence (%)		
	Apraclonidine 0.5%	Brimonidine 0.15%	Brimonidine 0.2%
Ocular			
Allergic conjunctivitis	NA	10-20	10-30
Blurred vision	1-5	—	10-30
Blepharitis	<1	1-4	3-9
Burning and/or stinging	5-15	5-9	10-30
Conjunctival blanching	1-5	—	3-9
Conjunctival edema	<1	1-4	3-9
Conjunctival follicles	<1	5-9	10-30
Conjunctival hyperemia	5-15	10-20	10-30
Conjunctivitis	1-5	1-4	—
Corneal staining/erosion	<1	<1	3-9
Dry eye	1-5	1-4	3-9
Eyelid erythema	<1	1-4	3-9
Foreign-body sensation	1-5	1-4	10-30

Lid edema	1-5	1-4	3-9
Pain	<1	3-9	3-9
Photophobia	<1	3-9	3-9
Pruritus	5-15	10-20	10-30
Tearing	1-5	1-4	3-9
Visual disturbance	<1	5-9	3-9
Systemic			
Abnormal taste	<3	<1	<3
Arrhythmia	<3	—	<3
Bronchitis	—	1-4	3-9
Dizziness	<3	1-4	3-9
Dry mouth	10	5-9	10-30
Fatigue/drowsiness	<3	<1	10-30
Headache	<3	5-9	10-30
Hypertension	—	5-9	<3

Abbreviation: NA, not available.

Physicians' Desk Reference for Ophthalmic Medicines: 2004. Montvale, NJ: Thomson Healthcare; 2003.

TABLE 10.7 — TOPICAL CARBONIC ANHYDRASE INHIBITORS USED IN THE TREATMENT OF GLAUCOMA

Generic (Trade) Name	Concentration (%)	IOP Reduction (mm Hg)	Dosage
Brinzolamide (Azopt)	1	3-5	1 drop tid
Dorzolamide (Trusopt)	2	3-5	1 drop tid

Abbreviation: IOP, intraocular pressure.

Physicians' Desk Reference for Ophthalmic Medicines: 2004. Montvale, NJ: Thomson Healthcare; 2003.

Oral Carbonic Anhydrase Inhibitors

There are several oral CAIs in current use (**Table 10.9**). They are indicated for lowering IOP in chronic OAG and secondary glaucoma, and in preoperative acute primary angle-closure glaucoma (PACG) when surgery is delayed.[3] Although oral CAIs are effective in lowering IOP, they are associated with systemic adverse effects (eg, fatigue, paresthesia) that frequently necessitate discontinuation of therapy.[5]

■ **Contraindications and Warnings**

Both acetazolamide and methazolamide are contraindicated in:

- Situations where sodium and/or potassium blood serum levels are depressed
- Cases of marked kidney and liver disease or dysfunction
- Suprarenal gland failure
- Hyperchloremic acidosis
- Patients with cirrhosis.

They are also contraindicated for long-term use in chronic congestive ACG. There have been rare fatalities from serious reactions to sulfonamides, including aplastic anemia, Stevens-Johnson syndrome, and fulminant hepatic necrosis.

■ **Adverse Reactions**

Oral CAIs may be considered as antiglaucoma agents reserved for later use due to their severe side-effect profile; up to 50% of patients cannot tolerate oral CAIs for long periods.[26] The common adverse effects associated with their use are shown in **Table 10.10**.

TABLE 10.8 — OCULAR AND SYSTEMIC SIDE EFFECTS OF CARBONIC ANHYDRASE INHIBITORS

Side Effect	Occurrence (%)	
	Brinzolamide 1%	Dorzolamide 2%
Ocular		
Allergic reaction	<1	10
Blepharitis	1-5	1-5
Blurred vision	5-10	1-5
Burning/stinging/discomfort	1-5	33
Conjunctival edema	—	1-5
Conjunctivitis	<1	1-5
Discharge	1-5	—
Dryness	1-5	1-5
Hyperemia (conjunctival)	1-5	1-5
Keratitis	1-5	10-15
Photophobia	—	1-5
Pruritus	1-5	<1

	<1	1-5
Tearing	<1	
Systemic		
Allergic reaction	<1	<1
Bitter or sour taste	5-10	25
Chest pain	<1	—
Dermatitis	1-5	<1
Dizziness	<1	<1
Dry mouth	<1	<1
Dyspnea	<1	<1
Headache	1-5	<1
Nausea	<1	<1
Urolithiasis (kidney stones)	—	<1
Urticaria	<1	<1

Physicians' Desk Reference for Ophthalmic Medicines: 2004. Montvale, NJ: Thomson Healthcare; 2003.

TABLE 10.9 — ORAL CARBONIC ANHYDRASE INHIBITORS USED TO CONTROL INTRAOCULAR PRESSURE IN GLAUCOMA

Generic (Trade) Name	Delivery Method: Concentration	Dosage
Acetazolamide (Diamox)	Tablets: 125, 250 mg	250 mg to 1000 mg/d
Acetazolamide (Diamox Sequels)*	Capsules: 500 mg sustained release	500 mg to 1000 mg/d
Acetazolamide sodium (Diamox)	IV: 500 mg vial	250 mg to 1000 mg/d
Methazolamide (Neptazane)*	Tablets: 25, 50 mg	50 mg to 100 mg tid
Abbreviations: IOP, intraocular pressure; IV, intravenous; NA, not available.		
* Available only in generic.		

TABLE 10.10 — COMMON ADVERSE EFFECTS ASSOCIATED WITH ORAL CARBONIC ANHYDRASE INHIBITORS
• Confusion
• Diarrhea
• Drowsiness
• Fatigue
• Hearing dysfunction or tinnitus
• Loss of appetite
• Malaise
• Nausea
• Paresthesias
• Polyuria
• Taste alteration
• Urolithiasis (kidney stones)
• Vomiting

Combination Agents

Many patients on glaucoma therapy are treated with more than one medication to control IOP. Although multiple medication regimens are commonly used, their inherent complexity creates therapy problems for patient compliance. Recently, fixed combination therapy (in which two topical ocular hypotensives have been combined in a single formulation) has become available. They provide the simplicity of monotherapy combined with increased efficacy from the additive effect of the two agents.

It is important to note that fixed combinations do not necessarily achieve the same degree of IOP-lowering efficacy as concomitant therapy with two separate medications. Each medication in the combination may effect the bioavailability of the other. Nevertheless, these fixed combinations hold great promise in controlling IOP while improving patient compliance. One such fixed combination, Cosopt, a combination of dorzolamide (2.0%) and timolol (0.5%), is currently available in the United States and worldwide.

■ Cosopt

Cosopt is indicated for the reduction of elevated IOP in patients with OAG or OH who are insufficiently responsive to β-blockers (ie, failed to achieve the target IOP level[s]).

Efficacy

In clinical studies, Cosopt, a fixed combination of dorzolamide (2.0%) and timolol (0.5%), given twice daily showed equivalent efficacy to the concomitant administration of dorzolamide (2.0%) given three times daily and timolol (0.5%) given twice daily in patients with either OH or OAG.[3,27] After washout of ocular hypotensive therapy, the IOP-lowering effect of Cosopt was significantly greater than that of either the dorzolamide (2.0%) or timolol (0.5%) components administered as monotherapy.[28] The overall incidence of adverse effects experienced by patients were comparable between the dorzolamide-timolol fixed combination and each of its components. While the proportion of patients who discontinued from the study due to clinical side effects were comparable between Cosopt and dorzolamide, it was significantly greater in the Cosopt group than in the timolol group.

Contraindications

Cosopt is contraindicated in patients with:
- Bronchial asthma
- History of bronchial asthma
- Severe obstructive pulmonary disease
- Sinus bradycardia
- Second- or third-degree atrioventricular block
- Cardiac failure
- Cardiogenic shock
- Hypersensitivity to any components of the product.[3]

Adverse Reactions

The adverse reactions to Cosopt are similar to those of the individual active agents, dorzolamide (0.2%) and timolol (0.5%). The most common side effects are shown in **Table 10.11**.

Cholinergic Agonists

The two most widely used cholinergic agents are pilocarpine and carbachol (**Table 10.12**). Pilocarpine has been available since the 1870s. Given the newer agents such as the PG analogues, topical CAIs, and α-agonists, the cholinergic agents are usually reserved for fourth- or fifth-line use. Nevertheless, they are quite

TABLE 10.11 — ADVERSE EFFECTS ASSOCIATED WITH COSOPT	
Side Effect	**Occurrence (%)**
Abdominal pain	1-5
Back pain	1-5
Blepharitis	1-5
Blurred vision	5-15
Bronchitis	1-5
Conjunctival edema	1-5
Conjunctival follicles	1-5
Conjunctival hyperemia	5-15
Dry eye	1-5
Ocular pruritus	5-15
Stinging and burning	Up to 30
Taste perversion	30

Physicians' Desk Reference for Ophthalmic Medicines: 2004. Montvale, NJ: Thomson Healthcare; 2003.

10

TABLE 10.12 — CHOLINERGIC AGENTS USED TO CONTROL INTRAOCULAR PRESSURE IN GLAUCOMA

Generic (Trade) Name	Concentration (%)	IOP Reduction (%)	Dosage
Carbachol (Isopto Carbachol)	0.75, 1.5, 2.25, 3.0	20	1 drop tid
Pilocarpine hydrochloride (Isopto Carpine)	1, 2, 4, 6	20	1 drop tid-qid
Pilocarpine hydrochloride (Pilopine HS)	4% gel	20	1/2-Inch ribbon qd

Abbreviation: IOP, intraocular pressure.

Modified from Shields MB. *Textbook of Glaucoma.* 4th ed. Baltimore, Md; Williams and Wilkins; 1998:387; and Kriegelstein GK. In: *Glaucoma.* London: BMJ Publishing Group; 2000:77-84.

useful in controlling IOP in the short-term and may be used long-term in conditions such as PACG associated with plateau iris configuration.

■ **Indications**

Cholinergics are indicated for lowering IOP in the treatment of glaucoma. Pilocarpine may be used in combination with other miotics, β-blockers, CAIs, adrenergic agonists, or hyperosmotic agents.[3] There is also a slight additive effect seen when pilocarpine is used in combination with the PG analogues (although the potential antagonistic effect of reduced uveoscleral outflow by pilocarpine is a concern in selecting this combination).

■ **Contraindications**

Miotics are contraindicated in situations in which pupillary constriction is undesirable, such as in acute iritis, or if there is hypersensitivity to any of the product components.

■ **Adverse Events**

Although pilocarpine can produce muscariniclike systemic adverse effects, systemic toxicity is rare with the usual doses of pilocarpine; it is normally seen only with strong miotics. The adverse effects of carbachol are more intense than those associated with pilocarpine. For this reason, carbachol is not usually prescribed for the long-term management of glaucoma.[7] Ocular side effects of these agents may be intolerable and result in a discontinuation rate of approximately 20% (**Table 10.13**).[5]

Nonspecific Adrenergic Agonists

Epinephrine is the principal nonspecific adrenergic agonist indicated for the treatment of OAG. It is

TABLE 10.13 — ADVERSE EFFECTS OF TOPICAL CHOLINERGIC AGENTS

Carbachol
- Ocular side effects:
  - Ciliary and conjunctival injection
  - Ciliary spasm/temporary decrease in visual acuity
  - Dimming of vision (miosis)
  - Stinging and burning
- Systemic side effects:
  - Asthma
  - Cardiac arrhythmia
  - Gastrointestinal cramping, diarrhea
  - Headache
  - Hypotension
  - Increased sweating
  - Salivation
  - Syncope
  - Vomiting

Pilocarpine
- Ocular side effects:
  - Burning or discomfort
  - Conjunctival vascular congestion
  - Dimming of vision (miosis)
  - Induced myopia
  - Lens opacity with extended use
  - Rare cases of retinal detachment
  - Reduced visual acuity in poor illumination
  - Superficial keratitis
  - Tearing
  - Temporal or periorbital headache
- Systemic side effects:
  - Gastrointestinal overactivity (rare)
  - Sweating (rare)

available as epinephrine and as the prodrug dipivefrin hydrochloride (**Table 10.14**).

Epinephrine has been used for >60 years as a standard for the treatment of glaucoma. However, its activity is less than that of timolol, and it is associated

TABLE 10.14 — EPINEPHRINE COMPOUNDS USED IN THE TREATMENT OF GLAUCOMA

Generic (Trade) Name	Concentration (%)	IOP Reduction (%)	Dosage
Epinephrine (Epifrin)	0.5, 1, 2	NA	1 drop qd or bid
Dipivefrin hydrochloride (Propine)	0.1	20-24	1 drop bid

Abbreviation: IOP, intraocular pressure; NA, not available.

Physicians' Desk Reference for Ophthalmic Medicines: 2004. Montvale, NJ: Thomson Healthcare; 2003.

10

with a range of ocular and systemic side effects that minimize its utility as a primary glaucoma therapeutic agent.[5]

■ Contraindications

Epinephrine compounds are contraindicated in patients with narrow angles or who have had an attack of PACG, since dilation of the pupil may precipitate such an attack. Another contraindication is a known hypersensitivity to any of its components.

■ Adverse Effects

Adverse effects are common with epinephrine compounds but occur less frequently with dipivefrin. The prodrug produces less burning and irritation with instillation, but once it is converted to epinephrine within the eye, it may have the same intraocular complications as standard epinephrine (**Table 10.15**).[29]

Hyperosmotic Agents

Hyperosmotic agents, administered orally or intravenously, are reserved for short-term emergency conditions such as acute PACG with extremely high IOP. Hyperosmotics are effective when the elevated pressure renders the iris unreactive to miotics such as pilocarpine. In rare instances, they are used to reduce vitreous volume prior to the initiation of surgical procedures. The rapid and dramatic IOP lowering seen with hyperosmotic agents may eliminate the need for glaucoma surgery in some cases. Side effects with hyperosmotic agents are serious, frequent, and sometimes fatal and are more pronounced with intravenous preparations. Hyperosmotics may precipitate renal or congestive heart failure and should be used with caution in patients with renal, cardiac, or hepatic disease. **Table 10.16** lists the various hyperosmotic agents and outlines their commonly seen adverse effects.[30,31]

TABLE 10.15 — ADVERSE EFFECTS OF EPINEPHRINE COMPOUNDS USED IN THE TREATMENT OF GLAUCOMA

Epinephrine
- Ocular side effects:
  - Allergic lid reactions
  - Brow ache
  - Conjunctival hyperemia
  - Cystoid macula edema
  - Eye pain
  - Follicular conjunctivitis
  - Headache
  - Reduction in endothelial cell thickness
- Systemic side effects:
  - Anorexia
  - Premature ventricular contractions

Dipivefrin
- Ocular side effects:
  - Allergic reaction
  - Blurred vision
  - Burning and stinging
  - Follicular conjunctivitis
  - Injection
  - Mydriasis
- Systemic side effects:
  - Arrhythmias
  - Hypertension
  - Tachycardia

10

TABLE 10.16 — HYPEROSMOTIC AGENTS USED TO CONTROL ACUTE ELEVATION OF INTRAOCULAR PRESSURE IN GLAUCOMA

Generic (Trade) Name	Concentration (%)	Dosage (g/kg)	Adverse Effects*
Glycerin (Glyrol)	75	1-1.5	Backache, cardiovascular overload, confusion, diarrhea, giddiness, headache, intracranial hemorrhage, nausea, pulmonary edema, renal insufficiency, vomiting[†]
Glycerin (Osmoglyn)	50	1-1.5	
Isosorbide (Ismotic)[‡]	45	1-1.5	
Mannitol (Osmitrol)	5, 10, 15, 20		
Urea (Ureaphil)	40 g/mL	0.5-2	

* Occur to different degrees with different preparations.
† More common with oral preparations.
‡ Recently discontinued by manufacturer.

Shields MB. *Textbook of Glaucoma*. 4th ed. Baltimore, Md: Williams and Wilkins; 1998:445-448; and Feiti ME, Krupin T. In: *The Glaucomas*. 2nd ed. St. Louis, Mo: Mosby; 1996.

REFERENCES

1. Alward WL. Medical management of glaucoma. *N Engl J Med.* 1998;339:1298-1307.

2. Geiser SC, Juzych M, Robin AL, Schwartz GF. Clinical pharmacology of adrenergic agents. In: Ritch R, Shields MB, Krupin T, eds. *Glaucomas.* 2nd ed. St. Louis, Mo: Mosby-Year Book; 1996:1425-1448.

3. *PDR Glaucoma Prescribing Guide.* 4th ed. Montvale, NJ: Medical Economics Company, Inc; 2002:1-99.

4. Schuman JS. Effects of systemic beta-blocker therapy on the efficacy and safety of topical brimonidine and timolol. Brimonidine Study Groups 1 and 2. *Ophthalmology.* 2000;107:1171-1177.

5. Schuman JS. Antiglaucoma medications: a review of safety and tolerability issues related to their use. *Clin Ther.* 2002; 22:167-208.

6. Epstein DL. Adrenergic agents: blockers and agonists. In: Epstein DL, Allingham RR, Schuman JS, eds. *Chandler and Grant's Glaucoma.* 4th ed. Baltimore, Md: Lippincott, Williams and Wilkins; 1997:137-152.

7. Gross RL. Current medical management of glaucoma. In: Yanoff M, Duker JS, eds. *Ophthalmology.* London: Mosby; 1999:12.24.1-8.

8. Shields MB. *Textbook of Glaucoma.* 4th ed. Baltimore, Md: Lippincott, Williams and Wilkins; 1998:440.

9. Brandt JD, VanDenburgh AM, Chen K, Whitcup SM, for the Bimatoprost Study Group. Comparison of once- or twice-daily bimatoprost with twice-daily timolol in patients with elevated IOP: a 3-month clinical trial. *Ophthalmology.* 2001;108:1023-1032.

10. Camras CB. Comparison of latanoprost and timolol in patients with ocular hypertension and glaucoma: a six-month masked, multicenter trial in the United States. The United States Latanoprost Study Group. *Ophthalmology.* 1996;103: 138-147.

10

11. Netland PA, Landry T, Sullivan EK, et al. Travoprost compared with latanoprost and timolol in patients with open-angle glaucoma or ocular hypertension. *Am J Ophthalmol.* 2001;132:472-484.

12. Nordmann JP, Mertz B, Yannoulis NC, et al, for the Unoprostone Monotherapy Study Group-EU. A double-masked randomized comparison of the efficacy and safety of unoprostone with timolol and betaxolol in patients with primary open-angle glaucoma including pseudoexfoliation glaucoma or ocular hypertension. 6-month data. *Am J Ophthalmol.* 2002;133:1-10.

13. Sherwood M, Brandt J, for the Bimatoprost Study Groups 1 and 2. Six-month comparison of bimatoprost once-daily and twice-daily with timolol twice-daily in patients with elevated intraocular pressure. *Surv Ophthalmol.* 2001;45(suppl 4):S361-S368.

14. Watson P, Stjernschantz J. A six-month randomized double-masked study comparing latanoprost with timolol in open-angle glaucoma and ocular hypertension. The Latanoprost Study Group. *Ophthalmology.* 1996;103:126-137.

15. Camras CB. Prostaglandins. In: Ritch R, Shields MB, Krupin T, eds. *Glaucomas.* 2nd ed. St. Louis, Mo: Mosby-Year Book; 1996:1449-1461.

16. Camras CB, Hedman K; US Latanoprost Study Group. Rate of response to latanoprost or timolol in patients with ocular hypertension or glaucoma. *J Glaucoma.* 2003;12:466-469.

17. Lima MC, Paranhos A Jr, Salim S, et al. Visually significant cystoid macula edema in pseudophakic and aphakic patients with glaucoma receiving latanoprost. *J Glaucoma.* 2000;9:317-321.

18. Schumer RA, Camras CB, Mandahl AK. Latanoprost and cystoid macular edema: is there a causal relation? *Curr Opin Ophthalmol.* 2000;11:94-100.

19. Data on file, Pharmacia and Upjohn Co; 2000.

20. Camras CB. CME and anterior uveitis with latanoprost use. *Ophthalmology.* 1998;105:1978-1981.

21. Eisenberg D. CME and anterior uveitis with latanoprost use. *Ophthalmology*. 1998;105:1978.

22. Thorne JE, Maguire AM, Lanciano R. CME and anterior uveitis with latanoprost use. *Ophthalmology*. 1998;105:1981-1983.

23. Katz LJ. Twelve-month evaluation of brimonidine-purite versus brimonidine in patients with glaucoma or ocular hypertension. *J Glaucoma*. 2002;11:119-126.

24. Nagasubramanian S, Hitchings RA, Demailly P, et al. Comparison of apraclonidine and timolol in chronic open-angle glaucoma. A three-month study. *Ophthalmology*. 1993;100:1318-1323.

25. Strahlman E, Tipping R, Vogel R. A double-masked, randomized 1-year study comparing dorzolamide (Trusopt), timolol, and betaxolol. International Dorzolamide Study Group. *Arch Ophthalmol*. 1995;113:1009-1016.

26. Lippa EA. Carbonic anhydrase inhibitors. In: Ritch R, Shields MB, Krupin T, eds. *Glaucomas*. 2nd ed. St. Louis, Mo: Mosby-Year Book; 1996:1463-1481.

27. Strohmaier K, Snyder E, DuBiner H, Adamsons I. The efficacy and safety of the dorzolamide-timolol combination versus the concomitant administration of its components. *Ophthalmology*. 1999;106(suppl 12):1-9.

28. Boyle JE, Ghosh K, Gieser DK, Adamsons IA. A randomized trial comparing the dorzolamide-timolol combination given twice daily to monotherapy with timolol and dorzolamide. *Ophthalmology*. 1999;106(suppl 12):10-16.

29. Shields MB. *Textbook of Glaucoma*. 4th ed. Baltimore, Md: Lippincott, Williams and Wilkins; 1998:403.

30. Feitl ME, Krupin T. Hyperosmotic agents. In: Ritch R, Shields MB, Krupin T, eds. *Glaucomas*. 2nd ed. St. Louis, Mo: Mosby-Year Book; 1996:1483-1488.

31. Shields MB. *Textbook of Glaucoma*. 4th ed. Baltimore, Md: Lippincott, Williams and Wilkins; 1998:445-448.

10

11 Comparative Clinical Trials/Primary Treatment Algorithm

As discussed in Chapter 10, *Medications for Glaucoma*, prostaglandin (PG) agents offer some unique advantages over β-blockers.[1] β-Blockers have been used as the gold standard for lowering intraocular pressure (IOP) in glaucoma and are still considered as first-line pharmacologic therapy for the treatment of glaucoma. However, there is a recent paradigm shift in treatment due to the multiple benefits of PG analogues:

- Greater efficacy when compared with β-blockers in lowering IOP over the diurnal cycle (both day and night)
- Intrinsic mechanism of action (increased aqueous outflow rather than decreased aqueous production)
- Increased potency (100 times greater than that of β-blockers)
- Improved systemic safety profile
- Simpler dosing schedules compared with conventional topical β-blocker therapy dosed bid.[1]

Recently, the Food and Drug Administration (FDA) approved the first-line use of one PG analogue latanoprost (Xalatan) in patients with open-angle glaucoma (OAG) and ocular hypertension (OH).

Systemic side effects and ocular tolerability are two major factors in selecting an IOP-lowering agent. Although the nonselective β-blockers have relatively few ocular side effects, there are a number of systemic side effects that are of concern—particularly cardiopulmonary effects. As a result, β-blockers may be unacceptable and contraindicated as first-line therapy in patients with cardiovascular or pulmonary problems. For younger patients who are more active, the increased lethargy and slowing of the heart rate that is associated with the use of β-blockers may preclude their use. In contrast, the PG analogues have little or no systemic side effects, although they do have unique ocular side effects. However, when balanced against their efficacy in lowering IOP, these ocular effects are usually tolerable.

Recently, there has been a distinct shift toward PG analogues as first-line therapy instead of β-blockers. However, the ocular side effects associated with the PG derivatives may render them unsuitable in some patients. These include a change in iris color that may occur in some individuals following long-term use. Such pigmentary changes most often occur in patients with green/brown, blue/gray/brown, or yellow/brown irides. Other ocular effects may include lengthening and thickening of the eyelashes and surrounding eyelid pigmentation. For patients in whom the above side effects are of concern, other hypotensive agents such as topical β-blockers, α_2-agonists, carbonic anhydrase inhibitors (CAIs), and anticholinergic agents, and combination therapy (ie, Cosopt [dorzolamide HCl and timolol]) may be used.

Comparative Clinical Trials

The PG analogues have been compared with β-blockers and with each other in a number of clinical trials. The following is a summary of the results of these clinical trials.

■ Trials with Timolol
Latanoprost
In clinical studies that compared latanoprost with timolol, latanoprost was shown to be equal or supe-

rior to timolol in reducing IOP. A 6-month random-ized, double-masked study had an 18-month, open-label follow-up.[2] Up to 277 patients were treated with latanoprost over 24-months, with 121 patients randomized to latanoprost (0.005%) once daily, and 128 patients selected to receive timolol (0.5%) twice daily during the 18-month follow-up. Both agents significantly reduced IOP (P <0.001), with a reduction in IOP of 34% for latanoprost and 33% for timolol after 6 months. These IOP reductions were maintained over the 24-month period. Systemic side effects were minimal. Ocular effects included iris pigmentation and ocular discomfort. Latanoprost administered once daily proved to be as effective as timolol given twice daily in patients with OAG and elevated IOP.

In another 6-month trial, Camras[3] found that both latanoprost (0.005%) and timolol (0.5%) significantly reduced IOP from baseline levels (P <0.001). Comparing 6-month with baseline diurnal IOP values (8AM, 12 noon, 4 PM), the mean IOP reduction achieved with latanoprost (–6.7 mm Hg) was significantly greater (P <0.001) than that observed with timolol (–4.9 mm Hg) (**Figure 11.1**). The authors concluded that latanoprost (0.005%) administered once daily is a more effective ocular hypotensive drug than timolol (0.5%) applied twice daily. They also reported that latanoprost is 100-fold more potent than timolol. No serious ocular adverse events occurred with either of these agents. In another comparative study, latanoprost (0.005%) applied once daily in the evening was statistically superior to latanoprost applied in the morning and to timolol dosed twice daily (P <0.001).[4]

The rate of response (in terms of IOP reduction) was recently reported for patients with glaucoma or OH who received either latanoprost (0.005%) once daily or timolol (0.5%) twice daily for 6 months.[5] The rate of response was determined based on mean diurnal IOP measurements at baseline and after 6 months

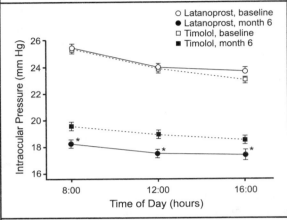

FIGURE 11.1 — DIURNAL EFFECT OF LATANOPROST AND TIMOLOL ON INTRAOCULAR PRESSURE MEASUREMENTS AFTER 6 MONTHS OF TREATMENT

Effect of 0.005% latanoprost ($n = 128$) applied once daily (at 8 PM) and 0.5% timolol ($n = 140$) applied twice daily (at 8 AM and 8 PM) on intraocular pressures measured at 8 AM, 12 noon, and 4 PM.

* Significant differences between latanoprost and timolol ($P < 0.001$). All values were significantly ($P < 0.001$) reduced from baseline.

Camras CB. *Ophthalmology*. 1996;103:138-147.

of treatment. Several criteria were used to define a "responder" including a specified percentage reduction of IOP, a specified mm Hg change in IOP, or a specified final absolute IOP level. Eyes with an IOP reduction ≤15% compared with baseline were classified as nonresponders. The results demonstrated that mean IOP reduction was greater ($P ≤ 0.001$) in latanoprost-treated patients versus timolol-treated patients throughout the entire course of therapy. Latanoprost produced a greater rate of response compared with timolol. In addition, a higher proportion of patients who did not initially respond became responders with continued treatment with latanoprost compared with timolol.

Bimatoprost

Bimatoprost (0.03%) bid and qd was compared with timolol (0.5%) bid in two randomized multicenter parallel-group, double-blind studies for 6 months.[6] Once-daily bimatoprost provided a significantly greater mean IOP reduction from baseline than timolol twice daily (P <0.001) after 6 months and at every follow-up. A target pressure of <17 mm Hg was achieved by 63.9% of bimatoprost qd patients compared with 37.3% of timolol patients (P <0.001). In addition to providing statistically and clinically superior IOP reduction compared with timolol, bimatoprost was safe and well tolerated.

Travoprost

A study evaluated the safety and IOP-lowering efficacy of travoprost (0.0015% and 0.004%) once daily compared with latanoprost (0.005%) once daily and timolol (0.5%) twice daily, in 801 patients with OAG or OH.[7] Patients were randomly assigned to receive travoprost (0.0015%), travoprost (0.004%), latanoprost (0.005%), or timolol (0.5%) for a period of 12 months. The results showed that both concentrations of travoprost were significantly superior to timolol in lowering IOP at all time points and visits. A response to treatment, defined as a 30% reduction in IOP or an IOP <17 mm Hg, was achieved in 49% of patients on travoprost (0.0015%), 50% of patients on latanoprost (0.005%), and 54% of those on travoprost (0.004%) vs 39.0% for timolol. Travoprost was deemed to be safe and effective with few ocular side effects.

■ Conclusion

In conclusion, the above studies have demonstrated that the IOP-lowering effect of latanoprost, bimatoprost, and travoprost is significantly greater than that of timolol. Moreover, these PG agents are safe and well tolerated.

Brimonidine

Three multicenter, randomized, double-masked, parallel group clinical trials compared brimonidine tartrate (0.2%) twice daily with timolol (0.5%) twice daily in patients with glaucoma or OH, and produced similar results.[8-10] At peak and at trough time points, both brimonidine and timolol provided significant decreases in IOP (P <0.001). All three studies found that brimonidine produced significantly greater reductions in IOP compared with timolol at peak effect. However, at trough effect, timolol produced a significantly greater decrease in IOP compared with brimonidine dosed twice daily (**Table 11.1**).

Clinical Comparisons Among Prostaglandin Analogues

■ Latanoprost vs Bimatoprost vs Travoprost

The recently completed Xalatan-Lumigan-Travatan (XLT) study was a 12-week, randomized, parallel-group clinical trial to compare the IOP-lowering effect and safety of latanoprost (0.005%), bimatoprost (0.03%), and travoprost (0.004%) once daily in the evening in patients with OAG or OH.[11] The study was designed with sufficient sample size to permit differences in IOP-lowering efficacy among the three medications of 1.5 mm Hg to achieve statistical significance ($P \leq 0.05$) with 80% power (ie, differences of <1.5 mm Hg would not necessarily achieve statistical significance). Decrease from baseline to week 12

TABLE 11.1 — BRIMONIDINE VS TIMOLOL: INTRAOCULAR PRESSURE REDUCTIONS AT PEAK AND TROUGH LEVELS

Study	Peak IOP Reduction (brimonidine > timolol)	Trough IOP Reduction (timolol > brimonidine)
Katz	$P < 0.0453$ at all times except month 6	$P < 0.001$ at all times
LeBlanc	$P \leq 0.007$ at weeks 1, 2 and month 12	$P < 0.001$ at all times
Schuman	$P \leq 0.04$ at weeks 1, 2 and month 3	≤ 2 mm Hg, difference not clinically significant

Abbreviation: IOP, intraocular pressure.

Katz LJ. *Am J Ophthalmol.* 1999;127:20-26; LeBlanc RP. *Ophthalmology.* 1998;105:1960-1967; Schuman JS. *Surv Ophthalmol.* 1996;41:S27-S37.

in 8 AM IOP (time of peak drug effect) was taken as the primary efficacy outcome for statistical analysis although measurements at noon, 4 PM, and 8 PM were also analyzed. In conjunction with recording of adverse events, masked investigators graded conjunctival hyperemia before the 8 AM measurement at each visit.

In all, 410 of 411 randomized patients from 45 US clinical sites were included in the intent-to-treat analyses (latanoprost 136, bimatoprost 136, travoprost 138). Baseline mean 8 AM IOP levels were comparable among the three groups: latanoprost 25.7, bimatoprost 25.7, and travoprost 26.5. At week 12, differences in estimated mean reductions (ANCOVA) from baseline for the 8 AM IOP reading, latanoprost 8.6, bimatoprost 8.7, and travoprost 8.0, were not statistically significant ($P = 0.128$) (**Figure 11.2**), and comparable mean reductions occurred at the other three time points. However, differences in ocular hyperemia were statistically significant. In comparisons between latanoprost and bimatoprost, fewer patients on latanoprost reported ocular hyperemia as an adverse event ($P = 0.001$), and the masked investigator hyperemia scores were also lower for latanoprost ($P = 0.001$). It should also be noted that efficacy of the three medications was not influenced by presence or absence of hyperemia during the trial.

Further analyses of the data were undertaken to determine whether there might have been a selection bias in favor of latanoprost super-responders in the XLT study. If that had been the case, then one would expect to find an enhanced response to latanoprost among the patients previously treated with a PG analogue (predominantly latanoprost). In fact, box plots of the appropriate subgroups showed no difference in response to any of the three medications between patients previously treated with a PG analogue and those not so treated.[11] Moreover, analyses of responder rates (in the ranges ≥15% and ≥20%), and percentages of

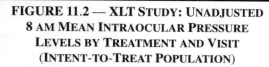

FIGURE 11.2 — XLT Study: Unadjusted 8 AM Mean Intraocular Pressure Levels by Treatment and Visit (Intent-to-Treat Population)

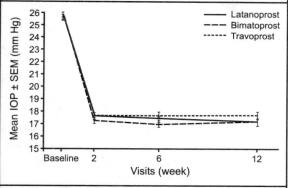

Abbreviations: IOP, intraocular pressure; SEM, standard error of measurement, XLT, Xalatan-Lumigan-Travatan.

Parrish RK, et al. *Am J Ophthalmol.* 2003;135:688-703.

patients achieving target IOP levels in the range 13 to 21 mm Hg revealed quite similar results for the three medications, and therefore no indication of a selection bias in favor of latanoprost[12] (**Table 11.2** and **Table 11.3**). In summary, the authors concluded that all three PG analogues were comparable in their IOP-lowering ability, but latanoprost exhibited superior tolerability.

■ Latanoprost vs Bimatoprost

In a randomized, multicenter, double-masked, placebo-controlled clinical trial, patients with primary open-angle glaucoma (POAG) or OH received bimatoprost (0.03%) once daily or latanoprost (0.005%) once daily or placebo.[13] Both bimatoprost and latanoprost provided significant mean decreases in mean IOP (from baseline) and in mean percent reduction from baseline (*P* <0.001). Bimatoprost provided a slightly greater re-

TABLE 11.2 — XLT STUDY: PATIENT RESPONDER RATES		
	Response Rate (%)	
Study Drug	**≥15% IOP Reduction**	**≥20% IOP Reduction**
Latanoprost	91.9	86.8
Bimatoprost	91.9	87.5
Travoprost	91.3	84.8

Abbreviation: IOP, intraocular pressure.

Parrish RK, et al. In Author Reply to: Noecker RS, et al. *Am J Ophthalmol*. 2004;137:211.

TABLE 11.3 — XLT STUDY: PERCENTAGE OF PATIENTS REACHING TARGET INTRAOCULAR PRESSURE LEVELS			
IOP Level (mm Hg)	**Latan (%)**	**Bima (%)**	**Trav (%)**
13	11	10	12
14	19	18	19
15	27	29	26
16	40	43	33
17	52	59	46
18	65	68	60
19	77	77	72
20	84	82	80
21	90	90	83

Abbreviations: IOP, intraocular pressure; Latan, latanoprost; Bima, bimatoprost; Trav, travoprost; XLT, Xalatan-Lumigan-Travatan.

Parrish RK, et al. In Author Reply to: Noecker RS, et al. *Am J Ophthalmol*. 2004;137:212.

duction in mean IOP than latanoprost, but IOP-lowering efficacy of both agents at 8 AM (primary outcome) was statistically equivalent (**Figure 11.3**).

Similar results were obtained in a randomized, multicenter, comparative, double-masked study that evaluated the safety and efficacy of bimatoprost (0.03%) or latanoprost (0.005%) given once daily for 3 months to patients with glaucoma or OH.[14] Both medications significantly reduced IOP from baseline at every time point ($P < 0.001$). Using bimatoprost, the mean IOP ranged from 17.4 to 17.6 mm Hg , and for latanoprost, the mean IOP ranged from 17.9 to 18.3 mm Hg. Target pressures of <17 mm Hg at 8 AM were

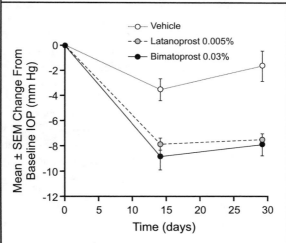

FIGURE 11.3 — REDUCTION IN INTRAOCULAR PRESSURE FROM BASELINE WITH ONCE DAILY DOSING OF BIMATOPROST OR LATANOPROST OR VEHICLE

Abbreviation: IOP, intraocular pressure.

DuBiner H, et al. *Surv Ophthalmol*. 2001;45(suppl 4):S353-S360.

11

achieved more often with bimatoprost than with latanoprost (53% vs 43%; $P <0.029$). At 3 months, bimatoprost achieved lower target pressures of ≤ 13 mm Hg, ≤ 14 mm Hg, or ≤ 15 mm Hg than latanoprost.

Both medications were well tolerated, with a low incidence of adverse events leading to discontinuation of the drug(s). The investigators concluded that bimatoprost was more likely to aid patients in reaching lower target IOP levels throughout the day, thereby potentially halting or preventing further vision loss. It should be noted, however, that there is a direct correlation between baseline IOP and the average IOP reduction with treatment. In both of these studies, the measured baseline mean IOP was higher for bimatoprost, which may explain, in part, the tendency for the greater reduction in IOP with use of this drug.[15]

More recently, Noecker and colleagues conducted a multicenter, randomized clinical trial (269 enrolled patients with OH or chronic glaucoma at 18 US clinical sites) to compare the IOP-lowering efficacy and safety of bimatoprost (0.03%) with latanoprost (0.005%) throughout a 6-month study period.[16] The primary outcome results were mean reductions from three baseline IOP measurements (8 AM, noon, 4 PM) at 1 week, 1 month, 3 months, and 6 months after initiation of treatment. Bimatoprost produced significantly greater mean IOP reductions from baseline than latanoprost at all three time points for each of the four intervals. At the sixth month, the bimatoprost excess IOP reductions were 1.5 mm Hg at 8 AM ($P <0.001$), 2.2 mm Hg at noon ($P <0.001$), and 1.2 mm Hg at 4 PM ($P = 0.004$). However, conjunctival hyperemia ($P <0.001$) and eyelash growth ($P = 0.064$) were more common in the bimatoprost-treated patients.

■ Latanoprost vs Travoprost

The efficacy of travoprost (either the 0.0015% or 0.004% concentration) was compared with that of latanoprost or timolol in a 12-month study by Netland and colleagues.[7] The PG agents were dosed once daily and timolol was dosed twice daily. Study results demonstrated that travoprost is comparable to latanoprost in lowering IOP in patients with OAG or OH. The mean IOP-lowering effect of travoprost (0.0015% or 0.004%) was comparable to that of latanoprost (0.005%). However, the mean IOP at 4 PM (from all visits pooled) for travoprost (0.004%) was 0.8 mm Hg lower than that for latanoprost ($P = 0.0191$) (**Figure 11.4**). Hyperemia, though relatively minimal in all groups, was significantly greater in both travoprost groups compared with the latanoprost and timolol groups. Finally, latanoprost and travoprost were reported to cause equal amounts of iris pigmentation.

■ Latanoprost vs Unoprostone

Latanoprost 0.005% taken once daily was compared with unoprostone 0.12% taken twice daily in an 8-week, double-masked, randomized, parallel-group trial in patients with POAG or OH.[17] Latanoprost reduced the mean IOP by 6.7 mm Hg compared with 3.3 mm Hg for unoprostone. The difference of 3.4 mm Hg was statistically significant ($P < 0.001$). This represented a 27.8% reduction in mean IOP for latanoprost and a 14% reduction for unoprostone. The response rate, defined as a 30% reduction in mean IOP from baseline, was achieved in 44% of latanoprost-treated patients compared with only 8% of unoprostone-treated patients. The study investigators concluded that latanoprost is significantly more effective than unoprostone in lowering IOP. Both drugs were well tolerated.

■ Summary

In summary, the above referenced studies demonstrate that in patients with POAG or OH, latanoprost, bimatoprost, and travoprost are comparable in IOP-

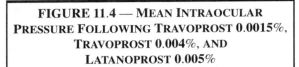

FIGURE 11.4 — MEAN INTRAOCULAR PRESSURE FOLLOWING TRAVOPROST 0.0015%, TRAVOPROST 0.004%, AND LATANOPROST 0.005%

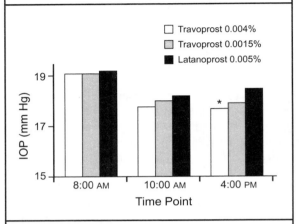

Abbreviation: IOP, intraocular pressure.

* Mean IOP-lowering efficacy of travoprost (0.004%) was significantly better than for latanoprost at 4 PM ($P = 0.0191$).

Netland PA, et al. *Am J Ophthalmol.* 2001;132:472-484.

lowering efficacy. These and other studies also indicate a high responder rate for these agents; relatively few patients fail to achieve IOP control with them. Response rates based on target IOP reductions do vary among studies and with the specific PG analogues being evaluated.[3,4,7,13,14,17,18]

In appraising the disparate results of the Parrish/XLT study compared with the Noecker study with regard to the IOP-lowering efficacy of latanoprost vs bimatoprost, it is important to consider the potential impact of lack of standardization of such studies. Regrettably, variables inherent in design, conduct, and interpretation of results of these randomized clinical trials may lead to apparent differences in outcome when the actual discrepancies may be minimal or even nonexistent. As Kaufman suggests, where the actual difference in efficacy between two drugs is slight, enormous sample sizes would be required to accurately pinpoint that difference, and divergent outcomes derived from lesser sample sizes could be due to chance alone or variations in patient populations (eg, receptor characteristics, rate of penetration in the case of topical prodrugs, etc). On the other hand, where the difference in efficacy is appreciable and clinically relevant, it is likely to be evident in nearly all studies despite the aforementioned variable factors.[19]

Persistency of Medical Therapy

While controlled clinical trials are undertaken to establish the efficacy and safety of medications, the results of these studies may not accurately reflect what can be achieved in routine clinical practice settings wherein patients are not preselected and care is not as carefully regimented. One important patient behavior not easily measured in controlled clinical trials is that of persistency of medical therapy (ie, time on therapy). This variable factor is especially critical in the treatment of a chronic disease such as glaucoma because inconsistent adherence to therapy may lead to wide fluctuations in IOP. In fact, variability and fluctuation over time have recently been reported to be significant risk factors for glaucomatous visual field progression in both the Advanced Glaucoma Intervention Study[20] and the Collaborative Initial Glaucoma Treatment Study.[21]

Persistency rates are not uniform across treatments for a given condition, and this variability appears to be related primarily to differences in efficacy and tolerability of medications.[22] In a retrospective cohort

177

study of a managed care database of approximately three million members, Reardon and associates evaluated persistency with specific topical ocular hypotensive agents, as reflected in prescription refill analyses in 28,741 glaucoma patients new to treatment (ie, monotherapy).[23] While persistency rates dropped off sharply during the first 90 to 180 days for all seven agents that were deployed, the latanoprost-treated patients maintained significantly greater persistency than patients treated initially with the other six agents (ie, timolol, betaxolol, dorzolamide, brimonidine, travoprost, and bimatoprost). It is important to note that the calculations of persistency relied on retrospective analyses of medication claims data, a method with several potential sources of error, such as incomplete records, non-assessment of reasons for discontinuing or changing therapy, lack of cost considerations, etc. Nevertheless, clinicians may wish to utilize comparative persistency rates as an important consideration in selecting among medications with similar pharmacotherapeutic effects.

Adjunctive or Additive Therapy

Adjunctive therapy is considered only when first-line medical therapy is inadequate in achieving the target IOP. In addition, it is only considered when another agent cannot be substituted to achieve the desired IOP. A common choice is the addition of another IOP-lowering agent to a β-blocker, such as timolol. Maximum tolerable medical therapy that may consist of as many as four or more medications (from different classes of ocular hypotensive agents) is often preferred by patients prior to consideration of laser trabeculoplasty and/or filtration surgery.[24]

In applying this stepwise additive therapy, drug safety profiles and risks to patients must be thoughtfully considered on an individual patient basis. Second, the financial cost of multiple medications may also be a major consideration for the patient.[25] Finally, patient compliance with a medication regimen must also be taken into consideration. Compliance may decrease with both increased frequency and complexity of maximum tolerable medical therapy. For example, a contemporary approach to a patient with inadequate response to a first-line β-blocker would involve the substitution of a potentially more effective PG agent (in place of the β-blocker) before resorting to additive therapy. This approach enhances patient compliance while minimizing the potential for cumulative side effects and drug interactions.

Unilateral Trials to Assess Efficacy

Unilateral, or one-eyed trials, allow evaluation of a particular drug's efficacy in lowering IOP. When possible, all medications should be administered initially in only one eye. The IOPs in both eyes should be assessed at the next follow-up visit. Given the variability of the diurnal IOP curve, the efficacy of the new agent can only be evaluated when compared with the IOP level of the contralateral eye. This comparison of IOP levels between the treated and control eye enables the clinician to identify and forgo use of ineffective agents, thereby minimizing the risk of unnecessary side effects, inconvenience, and financial cost to the patient.

A reverse unilateral trial can be performed by discontinuing a drug in one eye and then assessing the IOP effect. In this manner, an ineffective agent can be discontinued, while an effective agent can be retained. Reverse unilateral trials can also be enacted at any point during therapy to determine if adjunctive or switch therapy is required.

Other Current and Future Treatments

■ Alternative Medicines

Alternative therapies, such as herbal medicines, have shown considerable promise in treating a number of medical diseases and conditions. Ginkgo biloba, from the leaves of the maiden hair tree, inhibits platelet activating factor, has antioxidant activity, increases peripheral and cerebral blood flow, and offers neuroprotection (prevents glutamate neurotoxicity and neuronal injury). Ginkgo has been shown to improve ocular blood flow.[26] However, problems with spontaneous bleeding (eg, subarachnoid hemorrhage, subdural hematoma) have been reported in patients taking the compound.[27] Therefore, patients who take anticoagulants or who are at risk for intracranial bleeding should take ginkgo with extreme caution.

Bilberry acts as an antioxidant, inhibits platelet aggregation, and protects against reperfusion injury. Anecdotally, it was used successfully by World War II pilots to improve night vision.[27] However, there are no known published scientific studies of its effect on IOP or visual function.

In recent years, there has been a greater interest in the use of vitamins in the treatment of glaucoma. Vitamin C, a ubiquitous alternative therapy, has been shown to reduce IOP when given in massive doses, based on a hyperosmotic effect.[28] Oral doses of 2 mg per day have lowered IOP by 1.10 mm Hg.[29] Vitamin E has no effect on IOP but may be valuable as an adjunct to filtering surgery.

Marijuana cigarettes (2% concentration) reduce IOP by approximately 25% in approximately 60% to 65% of patients for about 2 hours.[30] However, smoking of marijuana plant material is ill-advised given its well-known toxic side effects. Topical forms appear to be ineffective and cause considerable ocular irritation.

Cannabinoids, compounds related to the tetrahydrocannabinol (THC) in marijuana, are under investigation.[31]

■ Neuroprotective Agents

Since glaucoma has been defined as an optic neuropathy, agents that afford neuroprotection by preventing or slowing retinal ganglion cell (RGC) death have the potential for halting its progression. In this respect, brimonidine has shown potential. Brimonidine has a high affinity for α_2-adrenergic receptors, which are present in the human retina.[32] Studies have shown that levels of brimonidine that are measured near the retina reach a sufficient level to bind to and activate the receptors responsible for neuroprotective activity.[33] Brimonidine has also been shown to be neuroprotective in animal models with chronic OH.[34,35]

Nitric oxide, which is present in human optic nerve heads, reacts with superoxide to produce a highly reactive free radical in human glaucomatous eyes.[36] Aminoguanidine, an inhibitor of nitric oxide synthase-2, has been shown to significantly reduce neuronal cell loss in animal models of induced glaucoma.

Memantine is another promising agent. It is an NMDA-type glutamate open-channel blocker. Neuronal damage may occur as a result of overstimulation of NMDA receptors in RGCs, caused by an excess of excitatory amino acids such as glutamate.[6] Memantine has been shown to preserve the visually evoked cortical potential and reduce RGC loss in animal models with experimentally induced glaucoma.[37]

■ Medications for Enhancing Ocular Blood Flow

Researchers and clinicians have postulated that compromised ocular blood flow, as a result of vascular insufficiency in the optic nerve head, contributes to the pathogenesis of glaucomatous optic neuropathy (GON).[38] Therefore, agents that enhance ocular blood flow and minimize damage caused by ischemia may act to prevent or slow the progress of GON. However, it is difficult to assess the effect of enhanced ocular blood flow on RGC deterioration or to determine whether relevant blood vessels are affected by therapeutic strategies designed to increase ocular blood flow. Nevertheless, there are several promising agents that have been reported to improve ocular blood flow with the potential to offer a vasoprotective effect against glaucomatous deterioration. Dorzolamide, a topical CAI, has been shown to increase retinal artery flow velocities in normal-tension glaucoma patients,[39] and topical verapamil increased retinal artery and optic disc capillary blood flow in normal subjects.[40,41]

Primary Treatment Algorithm

Information presented in Chapters 9, *Landmark Glaucoma Studies* and 10, *Medications for Glaucoma* make it possible to construct an algorithm for the primary treatment of OAG (**Figure 11.5**). The selection of medication choices in the algorithm was based on a myriad of factors including efficacy, ocular and systemic tolerability, persistency, ease of compliance, and mechanism of action. The inclusion criteria for applying this algorithm are:

- The patient is not currently on IOP-lowering medications
- A reduction in IOP of at least 20% from baseline and/or >4 mm Hg is required.

■ Option 1—Prostaglandin as Primary Therapy

Deployment of a PG analogue is considered acceptable if there is no contraindication due to such preexisting conditions as anterior uveitis, herpes simplex keratitis, or cystoid macular edema, and if the patient accepts the risk of possible ocular pigmentary changes. In that case, treatment may begin with a unilateral trial on latanoprost, the only PG agent approved by the

FDA for first-line use. If the desired IOP reduction is achieved, then simply prescribe bilateral treatment with latanoprost.

If the degree of IOP reduction with latanoprost is significant, but insufficiently effective, the next step consists of unilateral testing of a second agent superimposed on bilateral latanoprost, ultimately culminating in bilateral deployment of latanoprost and the additional agent. The preferred second agent would be timolol or another β-blocker (or Cosopt) if use of a β-blocker is acceptable. However, if β-blockers are either not acceptable or found to be ineffective and/or intolerable, the second agent would be a topical CAI (dorzolamide or brinzolamide) or brimonidine. In some recalcitrant cases, it might be advisable to try another PG analogue (bimatoprost or travoprost) in place of latanoprost.

If a PG analogue is not acceptable or latanoprost, when tested, should turn out to be ineffective (rather than insufficiently effective) and/or intolerable, proceed to Option 2.

■ Option 2—β-Blocker or Other Agents as Primary Therapy

When PG derivatives are not acceptable from the start, a β-blocker, if acceptable (ie, not contraindicated and not used in conjunction with a systemic β-blocker), usually timolol, would be the preferable first-line medication. A desired outcome of unilateral testing would result in bilateral β-blocker treatment. A significant, but insufficiently effective, IOP reduction would result in unilateral testing and bilateral deployment of a second agent, either a topical CAI or brimonidine (or even both in some cases), in addition to the β-blocker.

An ineffective and/or intolerable outcome of unilateral β-blocker testing would result in utilization of a topical CAI or brimonidine or both, or, if feasible, reconsideration of latanoprost. The same result would

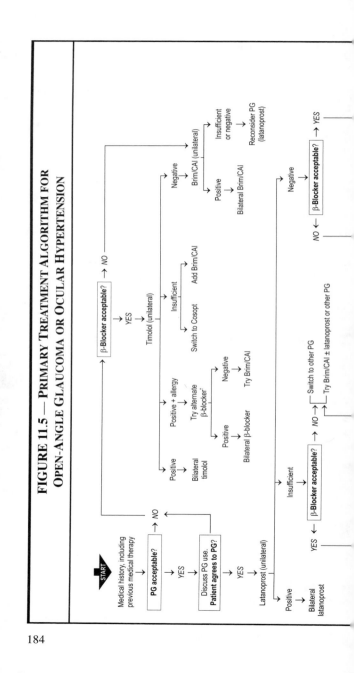

FIGURE 11.5 — PRIMARY TREATMENT ALGORITHM FOR OPEN-ANGLE GLAUCOMA OR OCULAR HYPERTENSION

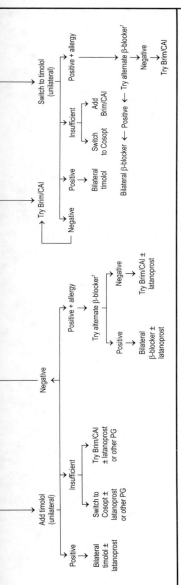

Abbreviations: Brim, brimonidine; CAI, (topical) carbonic anhydrase inhibitor; IOP, intraocular pressure; PG, prostaglandin.

Key: Positive = IOP reduced to target level and medication tolerable; negative = IOP not reduced and/or medication intolerable; Insufficient = IOP reduced (but not to target level) and medication tolerable; positive + allergy = for timolol: IOP reduced to target level and local allergy without systemic problem; ± = with or without an insufficient agent.

* No current medications, IOP inadequate, need at least 20% IOP reduction and/or >4 mm Hg reduction.
† Alternate β-blockers: carteolol, betaxolol, levobunolol.

Add timolol (unilateral)
→ Positive → Bilateral timolol ± latanoprost
→ Insufficient → Switch to Cosopt ± latanoprost or other PG / Try Brim/CAI ± latanoprost or other PG
→ Negative

→ Try Brim/CAI
→ Positive + allergy → Try alternate β-blocker† → Positive → Bilateral β-blocker ± latanoprost / Negative → Try Brim/CAI ± latanoprost
→ Negative
→ Positive → Bilateral timolol → Switch to Cosopt ← Positive → Bilateral β-blocker ← Try alternate β-blocker† / Add Brim/CAI
→ Insufficient

Switch to timolol (unilateral)
→ Positive + allergy → Try alternate β-blocker† → Negative → Try Brim/CAI

pertain if β-blockers and PG analogues were both deemed to be not acceptable at the outset; in that case a topical CAI or brimonidine would be prescribed on a first-line basis.

REFERENCES

1. Camras CB. Prostaglandins. In: Ritch R, Shields MB, Krupin T, eds. *Glaucomas*. 2nd ed. St. Louis, Mo: Mosby-Year Book; 1996:1449-1461.

2. Watson PG. Latanoprost. Two years' experience of its use in the United Kingdom. Latanoprost Study Group. *Ophthalmology*. 1998;105:82-87.

3. Camras CB. Comparison of latanoprost and timolol in patients with ocular hypertension and glaucoma: a six-month masked, multicenter trial in the United States. The United States Latanoprost Study Group. *Ophthalmology*. 1996;103:138-147.

4. Alm A, Stjernschantz J. Effects on intraocular pressure and side effects of 0.005% latanoprost applied once daily, evening or morning. A comparison with timolol. Scandinavian Latanoprost Study Group. *Ophthalmology*. 1995;102:1743-1752.

5. Camras CB, Hedman K; US Latanoprost Study Group. Rate of response to latanoprost or timolol in patients with ocular hypertension or glaucoma. *J Glaucoma*. 2003;12:466-469.

6. Sherwood M, Brandt J, for the Bimatoprost Study Groups 1 and 2. Six-month comparison of bimatoprost once-daily and twice-daily with timolol twice-daily in patients with elevated intraocular pressure. *Surv Ophthalmol*. 2001;45(suppl 4):S361-S368.

7. Netland PA, Landry T, Sullivan EK, et al, for the Travoprost Study Group. Travoprost compared with latanoprost and timolol in patients with open-angle glaucoma or ocular hypertension. *Am J Ophthalmol*. 2001;132:472-484.

8. Katz LJ. Brimonidine tartrate 0.2% twice daily vs timolol 0.5% twice daily: 1-year results in glaucoma patients. Brimonidine Study Group. *Am J Ophthalmol*. 1999;127:20-26.

9. LeBlanc RP. Twelve-month results of an ongoing randomized trial comparing brimonidine tartrate 0.2% and timolol 0.5% given twice daily in patients with glaucoma or ocular hypertension. Brimonidine Study Group 2. *Ophthalmology*. 1998;105:1960-1967.

10. Schuman JS. Clinical experience with brimonidine 0.2% and timolol 0.5% in glaucoma and ocular hypertension. *Surv Ophthalmol*. 1996;41:S27-S37.

11. Parrish RK, Palmberg P, Sheu WP; XLT Study Group. A comparison of latanoprost, bimatoprost, and travoprost in patients with elevated intraocular pressure: a 12-week, randomized, masked-evaluator multicenter study. *Am J Ophthalmol*. 2003;135:688-703.

12. Parrish RK, Palmberg P, Sheu WP. In Author reply to: Noecker RS, Dirks, Choplin N; Bimatoprost/Latanoprost Study Group. Comparison of latanoprost, bimatoprost, and travoprost in patients with elevated intraocular pressure: a 12-week, randomized, masked-evaluator multicenter study. *Am J Ophthalmol*. 2004;137:210-211; author reply 211-212.

13. DuBiner H, Cooke D, Dirks M, Stewart WC, VanDenburgh AM, Felix C. Efficacy and safety of bimatoprost in patients with elevated intraocular pressure: a 30-day comparison with latanoprost. *Surv Ophthalmol*. 2001;45(suppl 4):S353-S360.

14. Gandolfi S, Simmons ST, Sturm R, Chen K, VanDenburgh AM, for Bimatoprost Study Group 3. Three-month comparison of bimatoprost and latanoprost in patients with glaucoma and ocular hypertension. *Adv Ther*. 2001;18:110-121.

15. Eisenberg DL, Toris CB, Camras CB. Bimatoprost and travoprost: a review of recent studies of two new glaucoma drugs. *Surv Ophthalmol*. 2002;47(suppl 1):S105-S115.

16. Noecker RS, Dirks MS, Choplin NT, Bernstein P, Batoosingh AL, Whitcup SM; Bimatoprost/Latanoprost Study Group. A six-month randomized clinical trial comparing the intraocular pressure-lowering efficacy of bimatoprost and latanoprost in patients with ocular hypertension or glaucoma. *Am J Ophthalmol*. 2003;135:55-63.

11

17. Susanna R Jr, Giampini J Jr, Borges AS, Vessani RM, Jordao ML. A double-masked, randomized clinical trial comparing latanoprost with unoprostone in patients with open-angle glaucoma or ocular hypertension. *Ophthalmology*. 2001;108:259-263.

18. Watson P, Stjernschantz J. A six-month randomized double-masked study comparing latanoprost with timolol in open-angle glaucoma and ocular hypertension. The Latanoprost Study Group. *Ophthalmology*. 1996;103:126-137.

19. Kaufman PL. The prostaglandin wars. *Am J Ophthalmol*. 2003;136:727-728.

20. Nouri-Mahdavi K, Hoffman D, Gaasterland DE, Caprioli J. Intraocular pressure fluctuation is a risk factor for glaucomatous visual field progression in AGIS. American Academy of Ophthalmology Annual Meeting Program. Anaheim, Calif (November 17, 2003). 2003:134.

21. Lichter PR, Gillespie B, Musch DC, et al, and the CITGS Study Group. Intraocular pressure as a predictor of visual field loss in the Collaborative Initial Glaucoma Treatment Study. Anaheim, Calif: American Academy of Ophthalmology Annual Meeting Program; 2003:133.

22. Schwartz GF. Persistency and tolerability of ocular hypotensive agents: population-based evidence in the management of glaucoma. *Am J Ophthalmol*. 2004;137(suppl 1):S1-S2.

23. Reardon G, Schwartz GF, Mozaffari E. Patient persistency with topical ocular hypotensive therapy in a managed care population. *Am J Ophthalmol*. 2004;137(suppl 1):S3-S12.

24. Choplin NT. Advances in the medical management of glaucoma. In: American Academy of Ophthalmology, ed. *A LEO Clinical Update Course on Glaucoma*. San Francisco, Calif: American Academy of Ophthalmology; 2000:1-8.

25. Stewart WC. Maximizing medical therapy for glaucoma. *Rev Ophthalmol*. 2002;9:39-41.

26. Chung HS, Harris A, Kristinsson JK, Ciulla TA, Kagemann C, Ritch R. Ginkgo biloba extract increases ocular blood flow velocity. *J Ocul Pharmacol Ther*. 1999;15:233-240.

27. Rhee DJ, Katz LJ, Spaeth GL, Myers JS. Complementary and alternative medicine for glaucoma. *Surv Ophthalmol*. 2001; 46:43-55.

28. Virno M, Bucci MG, Pecori-Giraldi J, Cantore G. Intravenous glycerol-vitamin C (sodium salt) as osmotic agents to reduce intraocular pressure. *Am J Ophthalmol*. 1966;62:824-833.

29. Linner E. The pressure lowering effect of ascorbic acid in ocular hypertension. *Acta Ophthalmol*. 1969;47:685-689.

30. Green K. Marijuana smoking vs cannabinoids for glaucoma therapy. *Arch Ophthalmol*. 1998;116:1433-1437.

31. Jarvinen T, Pate DW, Laine K. Cannabinoids in the treatment of glaucoma. *Pharmacol Ther*. 2002;95:203-220.

32. Bylund DB, Chacko DM. Characterization of alpha2 adrenergic receptor subtypes in human ocular tissue homogenates. *Invest Ophthalmol Vis Sci*. 1999;40:2299-2306.

33. Kent AR, Nussdorf JD, David R, Tyson F, Small D, Fellows D. Vitreous concentration of topically applied brimonidine tartrate 0.2%. *Ophthalmology*. 2001;108:784-787.

34. Wheeler LA, Gil DW, WoldeMussie M. Role of alpha-2 adrenergic receptors in neuroprotection and glaucoma. *Surv Ophthalmol*. 2001;45(suppl 3):S290-S294.

35. WoldeMussie E, Ruiz G, Wijono M, Wheeler LA. Neuroprotection of retinal ganglion cells by brimonidine in rats with laser-induced chronic ocular hypertension. *Invest Ophthalmol Vis Sci*. 2001;42:2849-2855.

36. Sherwood MS, Brandt JD. Future scientific directions. In: American Academy of Ophthalmology, ed. *A LEO Clinical Update Course on Glaucoma*. San Francisco, Calif: American Academy of Ophthalmology; 2000:83-88.

37. Hare W, Woldmussie E, Lai R, et al. Efficacy and safety of memantine, an NMDA-type open-channel blocker, for reduction of retinal injury associated with experimental glaucoma in rat and monkey. *Surv Ophthalmol*. 2001;45(suppl 3):S284-S289.

38. Hayreh SS. Factors influencing blood flow in the optic nerve head. *J Glaucoma*. 1997;6:412-425.

11

39. Harris A, Arend O, Kagemann L, Garrett M, Chung HS, Martin B. Dorzolamide, visual function and ocular hemodynamics in normal-tension glaucoma. *J Ocul Pharmacol Ther.* 1999;15:189-197.

40. Netland PA, Grosskreutz CL, Feke GT, Hart LJ. Color Doppler ultrasound analysis of ocular circulation after topical calcium channel blocker. *Am J Ophthalmol.* 1995;119:694-700.

41. Netland PA, Feke GT, Konno S, Goger DG, Fujio N. Optic nerve head circulation after topical calcium channel blocker. *J Glaucoma.* 1996;5:200-206.

12 Primary Angle-Closure Glaucoma

Pathogenesis

In primary angle-closure glaucoma (PACG), resistance to aqueous humor outflow results from contact between the peripheral iris and the trabecular meshwork, thereby preventing aqueous from entering the outflow channels.[1] This type of angle-closure glaucoma (ACG) is considered primary when it is not secondary to some other ocular disorder. Crowding of the anterior chamber angle in PACG is almost always due to either pupillary block or plateau iris configuration, with the former mechanism accounting for the overwhelming majority of cases.[2] Pupillary block in PACG involves functional obstruction to aqueous flow from the posterior chamber through the pupil because of a shallow anterior chamber, which creates apposition of the posterior iris to the anterior lens surface.[3] Thus a pressure differential develops between the chambers, with slightly greater pressure in the posterior chamber. This pressure differential bows the peripheral iris forward into direct contact with the trabecular meshwork, thereby closing the angle and initiating the process of ACG (**Figure 12.1**).

Diagnosis

■ Acute Primary Angle-Closure Glaucoma

In acute PACG, there is a rapid increase in intraocular pressure (IOP) due to sudden blockage of the trabecular meshwork by the iris. This condition is characterized by:

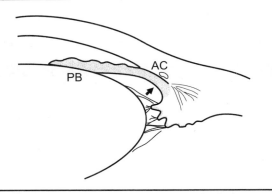

FIGURE 12.1 — PUPILLARY BLOCK GLAUCOMA

In pupillary block glaucoma, a functional block can be seen between the lens and iris (PB) that causes higher pressure in the posterior chamber (arrow). This results in a forward shifting of the peripheral iris and subsequent closure of the anterior chamber angle (AC).

Ritch R, Lowe RF. Angle-closure glaucoma: mechanisms and epidemiology. In: Ritch R, Shields MB, Krupin T, eds. *The Glaucomas*. 2nd ed. St. Louis, Mo: Mosby; 1996:801-819.

- Ocular pain
- Halos
- Blurred vision
- Nausea
- Vomiting.[4]

In all forms of ACG, measurements demonstrate that anterior chamber diameters, depths, and volumes are relatively smaller than those of normal eyes.[5] Additionally, it is critical to perform four-mirror indentation gonioscopy for an accurate assessment of a narrow or closed angle to distinguish between appositional and synechial closure.[6] There are numerous other signs that indicate the presence of PACG (**Table 12.1**).

Management Objectives

The objectives in the treatment of PACG are to:
- Rapidly abort the attack with medical treatment to minimize optic nerve damage
- Widen the angle configuration (with iridotomy) to prevent further closure
- Protect the fellow eye.

■ Medical Treatment

Medical treatment includes (see Chapter 10, *Medications for Glaucoma*):[4,7]

- Induction of miosis with cholinergic agents, such as pilocarpine, to draw the iris away from the trabecular meshwork. If the IOP is extremely elevated, pupillary block might worsen with these agents.

- Inhibition of aqueous inflow with β-blockers, carbonic anhydrase inhibitors, or α_2-agonists
- Hyperosmotics to rapidly reduce vitreous volume in an attempt to dramatically lower IOP, especially if the pupil is unresponsive to miotics.

■ Laser Treatment
Laser Iridotomy

Laser iridotomy—creating a full-thickness perforation in the peripheral iris—is the procedure of choice for PACG with pupillary block. This technique is easy to perform, except in some instances of unresponsive acute PACG, and causes few ocular complications. The procedure relieves pupillary block and usually opens the angle unless there are extensive peripheral anterior synechiae.[7] The advent of laser iridotomy, especially with the Nd:YAG laser, has obviated the need for surgical iridectomy in the majority of cases.[8]

Laser Iridoplasty

There exist situations in which an acute angle-closure attack is refractory to medical therapy and in which laser iridotomy cannot be performed (eg, corneal edema) or is not successful in rectifying the appositional angle closure. In these situations, argon laser peripheral iridoplasty may be used to open the anterior chamber angle.[9] In this procedure, low power, large spot size, and long duration laser burns are placed peripherally around the anterior stromal iris surface to create contractions in the iris tissue that pull open the angle (**Figure 12.2**).[10,11]

Ciliary Block (Malignant) Glaucoma

Malignant glaucoma is a term that was coined to signify an uncommon form of glaucoma that follows ocular surgery. It is characterized by a flat anterior

FIGURE 12.2 — ARGON LASER IRIDOPLASTY

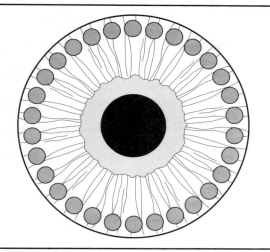

Stromal contraction burns are created around the periphery of the iris in argon laser iridoplasty.

Foster PJ, Chew PTK. Primary angle closure: management and prognosis. In: Hitchings RA, ed. *Glaucoma*. London: BMJ Publishing Group; 2000:162-170.

chamber in conjunction with markedly elevated IOP and is highly resistant to therapy.[12] The condition occurs in 0.6% to 4% of surgery associated with ACG.[13] A more contemporary term for this disorder, ciliary block glaucoma, is based on the concept that posterior misdirection of aqueous humor into the vitreous (due to a blockage involving apposition of ciliary processes, lens equator, and anterior hyaloid) causes obliteration of the anterior chamber with high IOP.[14,15] The characteristics of malignant glaucoma are listed in **Table 12.2**. This condition can be difficult to diagnose in its earlier stages before there is a rise in IOP.

Current medical treatment involves instillation of cycloplegic-mydriatic and ocular hypotensive agents.

TABLE 12.2 — DIAGNOSTIC CHARACTERISTICS OF MALIGNANT GLAUCOMA

- Occurs in eyes with chronic or acute PACG
- Usually follows surgical procedures for PACG such as iridectomy or trabeculectomy
- IOP is elevated
- May occur in pseudophakia
- Flattening or shallowing of central and peripheral anterior chamber
- Unresponsive to and possibly aggravated by treatment with miotics
- Usually responsive to cycloplegic-mydriatic and ocular hypotensive therapy
- Unresponsive to peripheral iridectomy

Abbreviations: IOP, intraocular pressure; PACG, primary angle-closure glaucoma.

Nichols DA. Malignant glaucoma. In: Sherwood MB, Spaeth GL, eds. *Complications of Glaucoma Therapy.* Thorofare, NJ: Slack, Inc; 1990:237-247; Simmons RJ. Malignant glaucoma. *Br J Ophthalmol.* 1972;56:263; and Chandler PA, Simmons RJ, Grant WM. Malignant glaucoma. Medical and surgical treatment. *Am J Ophthalmol.* 1968;66:495.

When ciliary block glaucoma proves refractory to medical therapy, the obstruction of aqueous humor access to the anterior chamber can be circumvented by means of laser or surgical intervention. Whenever feasible, an attempt can be made to either disrupt the anterior hyaloid with an Nd:YAG laser and/or shrink the ciliary processes by argon laser photocoagulation. If this attempt is not successful, lens extraction with posterior capsulectomy and/or pars plana vitrectomy should be considered.[12,16]

Plateau Iris

Plateau iris comprises a form of PACG without or with only minimal pupillary block. In this unusual condition, there is an atypical anterior insertion of the peripheral iris into the ciliary body such that the iris root angulates forward before turning centrally.[17] In addition, the iris plane is relatively flat in contrast to the forward bowing seen with pupillary block.[2] Following pupillary dilation, the peripheral iris bunches up into the angle and obstructs the trabecular meshwork.[4] In plateau iris–associated PACG, the central anterior chamber need not be quite as shallow as usually required for pupillary block–associated PACG to become operational.

REFERENCES

1. Hoskins HD Jr., Kass MA. *Becker-Shaffer's Diagnosis and Therapy of the Glaucomas*. 6th ed. St. Louis, Mo: The CV Mosby Company; 1989:214-215.

2. Shields MB. *Textbook of Glaucoma*. 4th ed. Baltimore, Md: Williams and Wilkins; 1998:249.

3. Lowe RF. Aetiology of the anatomical basis of primary angle-closure glaucoma. Biometrical comparisons between normal eyes and eyes with primary angle-closure glaucoma eyes. *Br J Ophthalmol* 1970;54:161-169.

4. American Academy of Ophthalmology. *Glaucoma. Basic and Clinical Science Course 2002-03*. San Francisco, Calif: American Academy of Ophthalmology; 2002:100-121.

5. Lee DA, Brubaker RF, Ilstrup DM. Anterior chamber dimensions in patients with narrow angles and angle-closure glaucoma. *Arch Ophthalmol.* 1984;102:46-50.

6. Forbes M. Gonioscopy with corneal indentation. A method for distinguishing between appositional closure and synechial closure. *Arch Ophthalmol.* 1966;76:488-492.

7. Ritch R, Lowe RF. Angle-closure glaucoma: therapeutic overview. In: Ritch R, Shields MB, Krupin T, eds. *The Glaucomas*. 2nd ed. St. Louis, Mo: Mosby; 1996:1521-1531.

12

8. Del Priore LV, Robin AL, Pollack IP. Neodmium: YAG and argon laser iridectomy. Long-term follow-up in a prospective randomised clinical trial. *Ophthalmology.* 1988;95:1207-1211.

9. Lim AS, Tan A, Chew P, et al. Laser iridoplasty in the treatment of severe acute angle closure glaucoma. *Int Ophthalmol.* 1993;17:33-36.

10. Ritch R. *Techniques of Argon Laser Iridectomy and Iridoplasty.* Palo Alto, Calif: Coherent Medical Press; 1983.

11. Ritch R, Liebmann JM. Argon laser peripheral iridoplasty. *Ophthalmic Surg Lasers.* 1996;27:289-300.

12. Ruben S, Tsai J, Hitchings R. Malignant glaucoma and its management. *Br J Ophthalmol.* 1997;81:163-167.

13. Nichols DA. Malignant glaucoma. In: Sherwood MB, Spaeth GL, eds. *Complications of Glaucoma Therapy.* Thorofare, NJ: Slack Inc.; 1990:237-247.

14. Weiss DI, Shaffer RN. Ciliary block (malignant) glaucoma. *Trans Am Acad Ophthalmol Otolaryngol.* 1972;76:450-461.

15. Shaffer RN, Hoskins HD Jr. Ciliary block (malignant) glaucoma. *Ophthalmology.* 1978;85:215-221.

16. Tsai JC, Barton KA, Miller MH, Khaw PT, Hitchings RA. Surgical results in malignant glaucoma refractory to medical or laser therapy. *Eye.* 1997;11:677-681.

17. Wand M, Grant WM, Simmons RJ, Hutchinson BT. Plateau iris syndrome. *Trans Am Acad Ophthal Otolaryngol.* 1977;83:122-130.

13   Secondary Open-Angle Glaucoma

Pigmentary Glaucoma

Pigment dispersion syndrome (PDS) is characterized by:

- Unusually heavy pigment dispersion on the corneal endothelium, often in a vertical spindle-shaped pattern (Krukenberg's spindle)
- Spokelike midperipheral iris transillumination defects
- Increased trabecular pigmentation.[1]

All these findings are due to liberation of pigment from the posterior iris epithelial surface in response to rubbing against the lens zonules. On gonioscopy, there is often characteristic posterior bowing of the peripheral iris (ie, reverse pupillary block). The Krukenberg's spindle is created by delivery of pigment granules to the cornea via aqueous convection currents and subsequent phagocytosis of pigment by the corneal endothelial cells.

When PDS is associated with glaucoma, the resultant ocular condition is referred to as pigmentary glaucoma. Deposition of excessive pigment in the trabecular meshwork outflow channels is believed to cause elevated intraocular pressure (IOP) and subsequent optic disc damage. The individual risk of developing glaucoma is approximately 25% to 50%, and its onset may occur as late as 15 to 20 years after initial presentation of pigmentary dispersion.[2] Those most commonly affected include myopic males between the ages of 20 and 50 years. Pigmentary glaucoma tends to respond favorably to laser trabeculoplasty (LTP) treatment, although the effect may not be long-lasting.[3]

Extensive variation in IOP levels is commonly observed in pigmentary glaucoma.[1] Patients may exhibit an exaggerated IOP response to steroid treatment. While laser iridotomy has been shown to alter the peripheral iris concavity that characterizes reverse pupillary block, the effectiveness of this intervention on the long-term course of pigmentary glaucoma has not been established. IOP levels sometimes improve or even normalize with advancing age (ie, burnt-out pigmentary glaucoma) as a result of decreased pigment shedding secondary to lens enlargement and correction of the reverse pupillary block.[3]

Exfoliation Syndrome (Pseudoexfoliation) Glaucoma

Pseudoexfoliative glaucoma is an open-angle glaucoma (OAG) that is secondary to the exfoliation syndrome (described in Chapter 7, *Pitfalls in Diagnosis: Primary Open-Angle Glaucoma*). The deposits of fibrillar material (histochemically resembling amyloid) occur throughout the anterior segment, including the lens, zonules, ciliary processes, corneal endothelium, anterior chamber angle, and anterior hyaloid.[1] A targetlike pattern of exfoliative material is often seen on the anterior lens capsule after pupillary dilation. In addition, peripupillary iris atrophy with transillumination defects can be seen. The trabecular meshwork is usually heavily pigmented, and an inferior pigmented deposition is often seen anterior to Schwalbe's line (ie, Sampoelesi's line).[4] Zonular weakness may lead to phacodonesis with shallowing of the anterior chamber and predispose affected eyes to zonular dehiscence, vitreous loss, and lens subluxation during cataract surgery.

Observed worldwide, exfoliation syndrome accounts for 15% to 20% of cases of OAG; it is the cause of >50% of identified cases of OAG in Scandinavian countries.[1,5] The syndrome occurs most commonly in individuals ≥70 years of age. Approximately 20% of individuals with exfoliation syndrome have glaucoma and elevated IOP at the time of diagnosis; another 15% develop increased IOP within 10 years. Moreover, 25% of patients who have unilateral pseudoexfoliative glaucoma develop the disease in the fellow eye within 10 years.[5]

The associated OAG is thought to be secondary to obstruction of aqueous flow and damage to trabecular meshwork as a result of the fibrillar material. The overall prognosis for pseudoexfoliative glaucoma is worse than that for primary open-angle glaucoma (POAG) because of its higher IOP and its greater resistance to medical treatment.[5] Although LTP can be very effective, its response may be short-lived; there is also an increased risk of IOP spike in the immediate postoperative period.[1]

Steroid-Associated Glaucoma

In susceptible patients, corticosteroid-induced elevation of IOP is possible from topical, subconjunctival, intravitreal, dermal, inhalational, or systemic administration of the agent. The IOP rise, as a result of decreased aqueous outflow facility, is observed in more than 50% of patients with POAG[6] (discussed in Chapter 7, *Pitfalls in Diagnosis: Primary Open-Angle Glaucoma*). However, the level of steroid-associated pressure elevation is quite variable in normal eyes. About two thirds of normal eyes have a low response to steroids, characterized by an IOP rise of <5 mm Hg. Approximately one third of normal eyes have an intermediate response, with an IOP elevation ranging from 6 mm Hg to 15 mm Hg. Only a small percentage (4% to 5%) of normal eyes are classified as high responders with IOP elevations >15 mm Hg.[6,7]

In general, the IOP rise occurs after the second week of steroid treatment, but it may occur after several months of treatment in low-responder patients. To reduce the risk of IOP elevation, the minimum required level of corticosteroid therapy, in terms of strength, duration, and frequency of use, should be adopted. Regular monitoring of IOP in patients who receive chronic administration of corticosteroids is warranted. Although the elevated IOP usually resolves within 4 weeks of discontinuation of steroid therapy, glaucomatous optic disc cupping may remain.[8]

REFERENCES

1. American Academy of Ophthalmology. *Glaucoma. Basic and Clinical Science Course 2002-2003*. San Francisco, Calif: American Academy of Ophthalmology; 2002:81-99.

2. Migliazzo CV, Shaffer RN, Nykin R, Magee S. Long-term analysis of pigmentary dispersion syndrome and pigmentary glaucoma. *Ophthalmology*. 1986;93:1528-1536.

3. Liebmann JM. Pigmentary glaucoma: new insights. In: *Focal Points: Clinical Modules for Ophthalmologists* (Vol 16, No 2). San Francisco, Calif: American Academy of Ophthalmology; 1998.

4. Barton K. Secondary glaucomas: classification and management. In: Hitchings RA, ed. *Glaucoma*. London: BMJ Publishing Group; 2000:196-213.

5. Samuelson TW, Shah G. Pseudoexfoliative glaucoma. In: Yanoff M, Duker JS, eds. *Ophthalmology*. London: Mosby; 1999:12.14.1-4.

6. Armaly MF. The heritable nature of dexamethasone-induced ocular hypertension. *Arch Ophthalmol*. 1966;75:32-35.

7. Armaly MF. Statistical attributes of the steroid hypertensive response in the clinically normal eye: I. the demonstration of three levels of response. *Invest Ophthalmol Vis Sci*. 1965;4:187-197.

8. Goldberg I. Ocular inflammatory and corticosteroid-induced glaucoma. In: Yanoff M, Duker JS, eds. *Ophthalmology*. London: Mosby; 1999:12.17.1-6.

14　Complications Following Laser Procedures

Most laser procedures have few sight-threatening complications. However, several of them deserve special attention since they may have serious consequences if left untreated. These include postlaser intraocular pressure (IOP) spikes and ocular inflammation.

Post-Trabeculoplasty IOP Spike

Intraocular pressure spikes most commonly occur 2 to 7 hours following argon laser trabeculoplasty. The same timetable is predicted after selective laser trabeculoplasty. If left untreated, the IOP elevation may cause further visual field loss in patients with advanced glaucomatous cupping.[1-4] In the majority of cases, the rise in IOP is <10 mm Hg above baseline IOP and lasts <24 hours with no permanent sequelae. In a small number of cases, however, the IOP elevation may be >20 mm Hg and sustained in duration.[2,5]

Eyes with an increased likelihood of post–laser trabeculoplasty (LTP) IOP elevation include those with advanced glaucoma (ie, severe trabecular damage) and exfoliation syndrome. Since it may be difficult to predict which eyes will have significant post-LTP IOP spikes, a postlaser IOP measurement should be performed 1 to 3 hours following the procedure, with measurement of the fellow eye as a control. Appropriate medical management includes, as needed, β-blockers, α_2-agonists, carbonic anhydrase inhibitors, anticholinergics, steroids, and oral hyperosmotic agents. Preoperative instillation of an α_2-agonist (apraclonidine or brimonidine) is useful to reduce the incidence and severity of these IOP spikes.[6]

Post-Iridotomy IOP Spike

Transient elevations in IOP are also commonly observed following argon and/or Nd:YAG laser iridotomy, especially in eyes with extensive peripheral anterior synechiae or underlying open-angle glaucoma. The inciting causal factor is a reduction in outflow facility, although aqueous inflow usually decreases.[7,8] Treatment with topical apraclonidine or brimonidine will markedly blunt the extent of this IOP elevation.[9,10] Failure to produce a full-thickness laser iridotomy may result in acute angle-closure glaucoma requiring emergency treatment.

Post-Iridoplasty IOP Spike

Marked elevations in IOP are common following iridoplasty and may pose a risk for the optic nerve.[11] These IOP spikes may be due to inflammation of the trabecular meshwork caused by shock waves from the laser burst or a blockage of aqueous flow through the trabecular meshwork by the release of particles from the iris. IOP spikes with the argon laser usually occur in the first hour following the laser procedure, and are generally transient—persisting for <24 hours—but in some cases, these IOP spikes may be sustained.[12]

Post–Panretinal Photocoagulation IOP Spike

Panretinal photocoagulation (PRP) is known to significantly reduce or eliminate anterior segment neovascularization.[13,14] By means of obliteration of retinal ischemic foci, PRP causes regression of rubeosis iridis and prevents severe secondary closed-angle glaucoma (if performed before synechial closure of the angle).[15] The etiology of the post-PRP IOP spike may be linked to development of postlaser ciliochoroidal effusions.[16]

Ocular Inflammation

Inflammation of the anterior segment—anterior uveitis—occurs frequently after laser procedures, including iridotomy, iridoplasty, and trabeculoplasty.[12,17] Transient iritis can result from breakdown of the aqueous-blood barrier following laser treatment. Occasionally, the inflammation can be severe enough to cause posterior synechiae formation.[18] In order to minimize the extent of laser-induced iritis, topical prednisolone drops four times daily for 3 to 5 days postoperatively may be instituted.

14

REFERENCES

1. Sherwood MB. Complications of argon laser trabeculoplasty. In: Sherwood MB, Spaeth GL, eds. *Complications of Glaucoma Therapy*. Thorofare, NJ: Slack Incorporated; 1990:89-99.

2. Weinreb RN, Ruderman J, Juster R, Zweig K. Immediate intraocular pressure response to argon laser trabeculoplasty. *Am J Ophthalmol*. 1983;95:279-286.

3. Krupin T, Kolker AE, Kass MA, Becker B. Intraocular pressure the day of argon laser trabeculoplasty in primary open-angle glaucoma. *Ophthalmology*. 1984;91:361-365.

4. Frucht J, Bishara S, Ticho U. Early intraocular pressure response following laser trabeculoplasty. *Br J Ophthalmol*. 1985;69:771-773.

5. Thomas JV, Simmons RJ, Belcher CD 3rd, Simmons RB. Laser trabeculoplasty: technique, indications, results, and complications. *Int Ophthalmol Clin*. 1984;24:97-120.

6. Cyrlin MN. Postlaser elevation of intraocular pressure. In: Epstein DL, Allingham RR, Schuman JS, eds. *Chandler and Grant's Glaucoma*. 4th ed. Baltimore, Md: Williams and Wilkins; 1997:470-471.

7. Krupin T, Stone RA, Cohen BH, Kolker AE, Kass MA. Acute intraocular pressure response to argon laser iridotomy. *Ophthalmology*. 1985;92:922-926.

8. Wetzel W. Ocular aqueous humor dynamics after photodisruptive laser surgery procedures. *Ophthalmic Surg*. 1994;25: 298-302.

9. Rosenberg LF, Krupin T, Ruderman J, et al. Apraclonidine and anterior segment laser surgery. Comparison of 0.5% versus 1.0% apraclonidine for prevention of postoperative intraocular pressure rise. *Ophthalmology*. 1995;102:1312-1318.

10. Chen TC, Ang RT, Grosskreutz CL, Pasquale LR, Fan JT. Brimonidine 0.2% versus apraclonidine 0.5% for prevention of intraocular pressure elevations after anterior segment laser surgery. *Ophthalmology*. 2001;108:1033-1038.

11. Schwartz LW. Complications of argon laser iridoplasty and coreoplasty. In: Sherwood MB, Spaeth GL, eds. *Complications of Glaucoma Therapy*. Thorofare, NJ: Slack Incorporated; 1990:113-121.

12. Ritch R, Liebmann JM. Laser iridotomy and peripheral iridoplasty. In: Ritch R, Shields MB, Krupin T, eds. *The Glaucomas*. 2nd ed. St. Louis, Mo: Mosby; 1996:1549-1573.

13. Little HL, Rosenthal AR, Dellaporta A, Jacobson DR. The effect of pan-retinal photocoagulation on rubeosis iridis. *Am J Ophthalmol*. 1976;81:804-809.

14. Jacobson DR, Murphy RP, Rosenthal AR. The treatment of angle neovascularization with panretinal photocoagulation. *Ophthalmology*. 1979;86:1270-1277.

15. Krupin T. *Manual of Glaucoma: Diagnosis and Management*. New York, NY: Churchill Livingston; 1988:163.

16. Tsai JC, Lee MB, WuDunn D, et al. Incidence of acute intraocular pressure elevation following panretinal photocoagulation. *J Glaucoma*. 1995;4:45-48.

17. Weinreb RN. Laser trabeculoplasty. In: Ritch R, Shields MB, Krupin T, eds. *The Glaucomas*. 2nd ed. St. Louis, Mo: Mosby; 1996:1575-1590.

18. Aslanides IM, Katz LJ. Argon laser trabeculoplasty and peripheral iridectomy. In: Yanoff M, Duker JS, eds. *Ophthalmology*. London: Mosby; 1999:12.26.1-4.

14

15 Complications Following Glaucoma Incisional Surgery

Adjunctive Antimetabolites

The most frequent cause of failure after glaucoma filtering surgery is filtration bleb scarring.[1] This excessive healing response may be due, in part, to the proliferation of fibroblasts and the production of collagen and glycosaminoglycans.[2] The antimetabolite 5-fluorouracil (5-FU) has been used adjunctively as a means of modulating wound healing in filtration surgery.[3] 5-FU inhibits fibroblast proliferation and retards against the associated bleb scar formation.[4] The pilot clinical study demonstrated that intraoperative and postoperative applications of 5-FU improve the outcomes of filtration surgery in refractory glaucomas.[5,6] Although it reduces postoperative intraocular pressure (IOP) and the need for antiglaucoma medications,[7,8] 5-FU also inhibits the growth of epithelial cells of the conjunctiva and cornea, and is associated with several undesirable complications including:

- Conjunctival wound leaks
- Corneal epithelial defects
- Thin-walled ischemic blebs
- Hypotony
- Suprachoroidal hemorrhage.

Mitomycin-C (MMC), another antifibrosis agent, is also highly effective in improving the outcome of filtering surgery.[9] Increased intraoperative use of MMC during glaucoma filtration surgery reflects its greater efficacy in inhibiting fibroblast growth when compared with 5-FU, thereby leading to still lower postoperative IOP.[9] However, use of MMC may cause prolonged hypotony with associated maculopathy, resulting in reduction of central visual acuity.[10] Moreover, MMC-associated (and 5-FU–associated) filtration blebs may involve a higher risk of early or late bleb leaks and late blebitis and/or endophthalmitis.[11]

Anti-inflammatory Agents

Corticosteroids are widely used to reduce postoperative ocular inflammation. They act nonselectively to control inflammation due to a variety of underlying causes.[12,13] For ocular inflammation, these agents can be applied topically, whereby they penetrate the cornea and sclera—in fact, this penetration is increased in an inflamed eye. Dexamethasone (0.1%) or prednisolone (1%), applied topically, is usually effective in anterior inflammation. Topical steroids have been associated with reduced wound healing and epithelial regeneration, which may lead to leaks at the site of surgical incision.

As noted elsewhere in this text, long-term use of topical steroids can produce elevated intraocular pressure (IOP) and steroid-induced glaucoma. Nonsteroidal anti-inflammatory drugs (NSAIDs) have come into use for anterior segment inflammation; they work by apparently reducing the breakdown of the blood-aqueous barrier.[14] It has been shown that the topical NSAIDs oxyphenbutazone, flurbiprofen, and diclofenac do not significantly increase IOP.[15-17]

Postoperative Bleb Massage

Digitally applied external ocular pressure, or digital massage of the globe, raises IOP, thereby forcing more aqueous through the sclerostomy site.[18] This manipulation of the globe results in broken external adhesions around the filtration bleb (thus increasing aqueous flow rate through the fistula) and increased area of external filtration (ie, larger bleb size). Digital pressure may also disrupt scar formation at the edges of the scleral flap and can be performed by the clinician and/or the patient.

Medical Management of Bleb Leak

Small and/or limited conjunctival bleb leaks may be managed medically in several ways. If the leak is situated close to the limbus, a sterile-bandage, soft contact lens soaked in antibiotic is an alternative to applying a moderately firm patch on the eye with antibiotic cover.[19] In addition, the short-term, concomitant use of aqueous-suppressant agents such as β-blockers or topical carbonic anhydrase inhibitors, may be helpful. Fibrin adhesives provide an alternative method of closing the bleb leak. To avoid the potential of infection with fibrin preparations derived from pooled human plasma, an autologous fibrin adhesive may be derived from the patient's own blood.[20] Autologous blood injections that incite an inflammatory response within the bleb to induce healing can sometimes be used successfully to treat leaking blebs.[21]

Management of Shallow Anterior Chamber

Hypotony and shallowing of the anterior chamber in the early postoperative period is not uncommon. This ocular condition usually occurs during the first several days following incisional filtration surgery and often gradually resolves over several weeks.[22] Intracameral injection(s) of a viscoelastic may help maintain the anterior chamber and reverse the ocular hypotony. In addition, intraoperative injections of

15

viscoelastic have been shown to reduce the incidence of postoperative shallowing—probably by preventing intraoperative hypotony.[23, 24] When hypotony is caused by leaks in the conjunctival flap, spontaneous closure may be obtained with a simple pressure patch. When there is excessive filtration secondary to a large filtering bleb, firm patching of the eye, possibly with the application of a Simmons shell, should be undertaken[25]; in some cases, revision of the trabeculectomy with tighter closure of the scleral flap may be required.

Management of Choroidal Detachment

Postoperative hypotony may contribute to serous choroidal detachment,[26] which may prolong the duration of hypotony. If they are limited in size, choroidal detachments do not impact the long-term outcomes of trabeculectomy.[27] It may become necessary to drain a choroidal detachment if the anterior chamber shallows substantially or if choroidal hemorrhage is a possibility.[28]

REFERENCES

1 .   Maumenee AE. External filtering operations for glaucoma: the mechanism of function and failure. *Trans Am Ophthalmol Soc*. 1960;58:319.

2.   Addicks EM, Quigley HA, Green WR, Robin AL. Histologic characteristics of filtering blebs in glaucomatous eyes. *Arch Ophthalmol*. 1983;101:795-798.

3.   Fluorouracil Filtering Surgery Study Group. Three-year follow-up of the Fluorouracil Filtering Surgery Study. *Am J Ophthalmol*. 1993;115:82-92.

4.   Krupin T. *Manual of Glaucoma: Diagnosis and Management*. New York, NY: Churchill Livingston; 1988:219.

5.   Heuer DK, Parrish RK, Gressel MG, et al. 5-Fluorouracil and glaucoma filtering surgery. III. Intermediate follow-up of a pilot study. *Ophthalmology*. 1986;93:1537-1546.

6. Heuer DK, Parrish RK, Gressel MG, Hodapp E, Palmberg PF, Anderson DR. 5-Fluorouracil and glaucoma filtering surgery. II. A pilot study. *Ophthalmology*. 1984;91:384-394.

7. Liebmann JM, Ritch R, Marmor M, Nunez J, Wolner B. Initial 5-fluorouracil in uncomplicated glaucoma. *Ophthalmology*. 1991;98:1036-1041.

8. Goldenfeld M, Krupin T, Ruderman JM, et al. 5-Fluorouracil in initial trabeculectomy. A prospective, randomized, multicenter study. *Ophthalmology*. 1994;101:1024-1029.

9. Skuta GL, Beeson CC, Higginbothom EJ, et al. Intraoperative mitomycin versus postoperative 5-fluorouracil in high-risk glaucoma filtering surgery. *Ophthalmology*. 1992;99:438-444.

10. Costa VP, Wilson RP, Moster MR, Schmidt CM, Gandham S. Hypotony maculopathy following the use of topical mitomycin C in glaucoma filtration surgery. *Ophthalmic Surg*. 1993;24:389-394.

11. Sherwood MB. New approaches to surgical management of glaucoma. In: American Academy of Ophthalmology, ed. *A LEO Clinical Update Course on Glaucoma*. San Francisco, Calif: American Academy of Ophthalmology; 2000:45-51.

12. Krupin T, Feitl, Karalekas D. Glaucoma associated with uveitis. In: Ritch R, Shields MB, Krupin T, eds. *The Glaucomas*. 2nd ed. St. Louis, Mo: Mosby; 1996:1225-1258.

13. Simmons ST. Medical management of wound healing in filtration surgery and its complications. In: Sherwood MB, Spaeth GL, eds. *Complications of Glaucoma Therapy*. Thorofare, NJ: Slack Incorporated; 1990:181-187.

14. Shields MB. *Textbook of Glaucoma*. 4th ed. Baltimore, Md: Williams and Wilkins; 1998:326.

15. Wilhemi E. Experimental and clinical investigation of a non-hormonal anti-inflammatory eye ointment. *Ophthalmic Res*. 1973;5:253.

16. Gieser DK, Hodapp E, Goldberg I, Kass MA, Becker B. Flurbiprofen and intraocular pressure. *Ann Ophthalmol*. 1981;13:831-833.

17. Strelow SA, Sherwood MB, Broncato LJB, et al. The effect of diclofenac sodium ophthalmic solution on intraocular pressure following cataract extraction. *Ophthalmic Surg*. 1992;23:170-175.

15

18. Krupin T. *Manual of Glaucoma: Diagnosis and Management*. New York, NY: Churchill Livingston; 1988:221.

19. Sherwood MB. Complications and management of large cystic blebs. In: Sherwood MB, Spaeth GL, eds. *Complications of Glaucoma Therapy*. Thorofare, NJ: Slack Incorporated; 1990:283-299.

20. Siedentop KH, Harris DM, Sanchez B. Autologous fibrin tissue adhesive. *Laryngoscope*. 1985;95:1074-1076.

21. Smith MF, Magauran R, Doyle JW. Treatment of post-filtration bleb leak by bleb injection of autologous blood. *Ophthalmic Surg*. 1994;25:636-637.

22. Kao SF, Lichter PR, Musch DC. Anterior chamber depth following filtration surgery. *Ophthalmic Surg*. 1989;20:332-336.

23. Wand M. Intraoperative intracameral viscoelastic agent in the prevention of postfiltration flat anterior chamber. *J Glaucoma*. 1994;3:101.

24. Wand M. Viscoelastic agent and the prevention of post-filtration flat anterior chamber. *Ophthalmic Surg*. 1988;19:523-524.

25. Shields MB. *Textbook of Glaucoma*. 4th ed. Baltimore, Md: Williams and Wilkins; 1998:521-522.

26. Brubaker RF, Pederson JE. Ciliochoroidal detachment. *Surv Ophthalmol*. 1983;27:281-289.

27. Stewart WC, Crinkley CM. Influence of serous suprachoroidal detachments on the results of trabeculectomy surgery. *Acta Ophthalmol (Copenh)*. 1994;72:309-314.

28. Fourman S. Management of cornea-lens touch after filtering surgery for glaucoma. *Ophthalmology*. 1990;97:424-428.

16   When Medical Therapy Is Insufficient

In the United States, medical therapy with ocular antihypertensive agents is the primary treatment for primary open-angle glaucoma (POAG). In a significant number of patients, combination therapy (either concomitantly or with fixed-combination agents) is often needed to reach target intraocular pressure (IOP) levels (see Chapter 11, *Comparative Clinical Trials/ Primary Treatment Algorithm*, under *Adjunctive or Additive Therapy*). For advanced glaucoma that is difficult to control, maximum tolerable medical therapy often involves concurrent use of three to four ocular hypotensive agents, but under special circumstances (eg, after failed surgery), there might be as many as five. Each of the five classes of antiglaucoma medications has a distinct mechanism of action which, in turn, lowers IOP by one or more of three pathways, namely:

- Reduction of aqueous production
- Increase of conventional outflow facility
- Increase of nonconventional, or uveoscleral, outflow (see Chapter 8, *Treatment Modalities: The Basis of Glaucoma Therapy* under *Combining Medical Therapies—Additive or Synergistic Mechanisms of Action*, and **Table 8.2**, **Table 8.3**, and **Table 8.6**).

Nevertheless, the glaucoma may remain refractory from either of two perspectives:

- Target IOP is not achieved
- Target IOP is achieved, but there is still evidence of glaucomatous progression.

In these cases, laser or surgical intervention should be considered.

Laser vs Surgical Considerations

■ **Trabeculoplasty**

When POAG is refractory to medical treatment, the choice of either laser or incisional treatment needs to be made based on the target IOP set for the patient. Either argon laser trabeculoplasty (ALT) or selective laser trabeculoplasty may be strongly considered as the next step, since both are less invasive and have fewer postoperative complications than more invasive filtration surgery.

In the majority of cases, ALT will provide a 20% to 30% reduction in baseline IOP (6 to 9 mm Hg)[1,2], with continuation of intensive antiglaucoma medical therapy. However, the simplicity and short-term efficacy of IOP reduction by ALT (in 85% of treated eyes)[3] must be balanced against the high tendency for loss of IOP control over time—20% after 1 year, 50% to 60% after 4 years, and 70% after 10 years.[4] Moreover, the reduction in IOP achieved with laser trabeculoplasty (LTP) may not be sufficient for a patient with markedly elevated IOP—eg, if a patient has an IOP of 35 mm Hg and the target pressure is 15 mm Hg, a reduction of 20 mm Hg may not realistically be achieved by this technique.[1,2] Therefore, eyes with markedly elevated IOP(s), continued progression of glaucomatous optic nerve damage, or loss of IOP control after previous trabeculoplasty may warrant the use of glaucoma filtration surgery (eg, trabeculectomy), rather than LTP, as the first intervention.

■ **Glaucoma Filtration Surgery**

Trabeculectomy has a success rate (in achieving the desired IOP reduction) of approximately 80% to 90% during the first year or so. Its long-term survival rate is approximately 70% (after 5 years) without the need for additional medication.[5,6] Complications associated with trabeculectomy include:

- Early complications:
  - Intraocular hemorrhage
  - Inflammation
  - Hypotony
  - Choroidal or uveal effusion
  - Leaking bleb
  - Endophthalmitis
  - Malignant glaucoma
- Late complications:
  - Lens opacities and cataract
  - Leaking bleb
  - Endophthalmitis
  - Loss of vision.[7]

Over the past decade, penetrating filtration surgery (ie, trabeculectomy) has been made safer and more effective with the incorporation of antimetabolite use and laser suture lysis/releasable sutures.[8] However, nonpenetrating filtration surgery (eg, viscocanalostomy, deep sclerectomy), glaucoma tube shunt surgery, and cyclodestructive procedures should also be considered as alternative surgical options (see Chapter 8, *Treatment Modalities: The Basis of Glaucoma Therapy*).

16

REFERENCES

1. Shingleton BJ, Richter CU, Bellows AR, Hutchinson BT, Glynn RJ. Long-term efficacy of argon laser trabeculoplasty. *Ophthalmology*. 1987;94:1513-1518.

2. Wise JB, Witter SL. Argon laser therapy for open-angle glaucoma. A pilot study. *Arch Ophthalmol*. 1979;97:319-322.

3. Migdal C. Laser treatment of primary open angle glaucoma. In: Hitchings RA, ed. *Glaucoma*. London: BMJ Publishing Group; 2000:85-90.

4. Schuman JS. New lasers for treating glaucoma. In: American Academy of Ophthalmology, ed. *A LEO Clinical Update Course on Glaucoma*. San Francisco, Calif: American Academy of Ophthalmology; 2000:23-25.

5. Mills KB. Trabeculectomy: a retrospective long-term follow-up of 444 cases. *Br J Ophthalmol*. 1981;65:790-795.

6. Watson PG, Grierson I. The place of trabeculectomy in the treatment of glaucoma. *Ophthalmology*. 1981;88:175-196.

7. Bechetoille A, Hitchings RA. Glaucoma surgery. In: Hitchings RA, ed. *Glaucoma*. London: BMJ Publishing Group; 2000;98:91-105.

8. Samuelson TW. Non-penetrating filtration surgery. In: American Academy of Ophthalmology, ed. *A LEO Clinical Update Course on Glaucoma*. San Francisco, Calif: American Academy of Ophthalmology; 2000.

17 Refractory Glaucoma

The term "refractory glaucoma" refers to those entities that are usually difficult to manage with conventional medical therapy. Several conditions warrant discussion since they are commonly encountered and are often refractory to medical treatment. These include:

- Glaucoma associated with epithelial downgrowth
- Glaucoma associated with inflammation (ie, uveitic glaucoma)
- Glaucoma associated with trauma
- Neovascular glaucoma.

Epithelial Downgrowth

Epithelial downgrowth (also called epithelial ingrowth) occurs most commonly following either trauma to the eye or ocular surgery (eg, cataract surgery).[1] In this condition, an epithelial membrane spreads into the eye through a penetrating wound, onto the corneal endothelium, and throughout the anterior chamber, including the iris and trabecular meshwork. The presenting signs and symptoms include:

- Persistent, low-grade postoperative inflammation, as well as conjunctival injection
- Photophobia
- Ocular discomfort
- Aqueous humor cells
- Translucent membrane on the corneal endothelium.[1,2]

The diagnosis can be established by argon laser photocoagulation of the iris, which produces white burns in areas covered by epithelium, or by microscopic detection of epithelial cells in aqueous humor specimens obtained via paracentesis. The long-term ocular sequelae include recalcitrant corneal edema and severe secondary closed-angle glaucoma. Although medical therapy may be instituted initially, severe recalcitrant cases may require either glaucoma filtration or tube-shunt surgery. Fortunately, the incidence of epithelial downgrowth is declining, in part due to the newer, smaller incisions employed in modern cataract surgery.[3]

Glaucoma Associated With Inflammation

■ Uveitis

Inflammation of the uveal tract and corneal endothelium can reduce aqueous inflow and/or obstruct trabecular outflow with resultant decreases or increases in intraocular pressure (IOP). When outflow obstruction is predominant, the persistent elevation in IOP can lead to glaucomatous optic atrophy.[4] Uveitic glaucoma may become recalcitrant to intensive medical therapy due to the following factors:

- Clogging of trabecular meshwork by increased protein levels, inflammatory cells, or cellular debris[5]
- Destruction and scarring of the trabecular meshwork collagen and beams[6]
- Scleritis secondary to the uveitis that may lead to scarring and fibrosis of the scleral outflow channels.[7,8]

Recalcitrant iridocyclitis may lead to secondary open-angle glaucoma (OAG) or secondary closed-angle glaucoma. The secondary OAG may result from obstruction of the trabecular meshwork by cellular exudates and inflammation of the endothelial cells lining the trabecular columns.[9] Gonioscopic evaluation may reveal subtle precipitates on the trabecular meshwork. On the other hand, the secondary closed-angle glaucoma may result from chronic inflammation with formation of peripheral anterior synechiae (PAS) or posterior synechiae with pupillary block and iris bombé.[10]

■ Herpes Simplex and Herpes Zoster

The most common type of keratouveitis with elevated IOP leading to glaucomatous damage is that caused by herpes simplex.[11,12] The keratouveitis caused by herpes zoster may also result in glaucoma.[13] Treatment of herpes virus–associated keratouveitis involves careful management of the ocular inflammation and glaucoma with corticosteroids, cycloplegics, and (non–inflammatory-provoking) ocular antihypertensive medications that reduce aqueous inflow, in conjunction with acyclovir.[14,15]

Glaucoma Associated With Trauma

The glaucomas associated with ocular trauma most commonly result from hyphema and/or angle recession (cleavage), a tear in the ciliary body between the longitudinal and circular muscle fibers. Hyphema, a frequent sequela of blunt trauma to the eye,[16] may provoke an acute elevation of IOP by clogging the trabecular meshwork with red blood cells. The degree of IOP elevation usually depends on the extent of the hemorrhage.[17] Angle recession—which occurs in up to 94% of patients experiencing ocular trauma—may lead to delayed-onset elevated IOP and an increased risk for glaucoma long after the injury.[18,19] Rebleeding, a serious complication of hyphema, is associated with an increased risk for acute glaucoma—up to 33% in patients who rebleed, and 100% in patients with total (eight-ball) hyphema.[20-22]

17

Neovascular Glaucoma

Neovascular glaucoma is characterized by neovascularization of the iris and angle. Such anterior segment neovascularization occurs as a result of retinal ischemia in a number of disorders with diabetic retinopathy, central retinal vein occlusion, and carotid occlusive disease being the most common causes.[23] Among the other causes of neovascular glaucoma are inflammatory diseases, such as chronic uveitis and intraocular neoplasms (which, if present, must not be overlooked). In all of these conditions, a fibrovascular membrane overgrows the iris and trabecular meshwork, after which it contracts to form PAS resulting in partial or total synechial closure of the anterior chamber angle. During early stages of the disease, the fibrovascular membrane itself blocks the trabecular meshwork leading to an open-angle type of glaucoma. With the development of PAS, the resultant secondary closed-angle glaucoma often leads to loss of vision. The current standard of care includes panretinal laser photocoagulation to curtail neovascularization with subsequent control of increased IOP by means of medical and/or surgical therapy.[23]

Based on an extensive review of the published literature,[23] **Figure 17.1** represents a proposed management algorithm for the treatment of patients with rubeosis and angle neovascularization. For eyes with useful vision, this algorithm focuses on identification and effective treatment of the underlying cause of rubeosis, which in most cases is retinal ischemia. For patients in whom adequate laser PRP treatment cannot be achieved, consideration should be given to aggressive retinal ablation by means of pars plana vitectomy with endolaser. Alternative methods, such as diode laser retinopexy and panretinal cryotherapy, should be reserved for patients unable to undergo vitreoretinal surgery (and eyes with little or no visual potential). Following cessation of neovascularization by means of either laser PRP, vitrectomy with endolaser, or an alternate method of panretinal ablation, it is essential to deal with the residual glaucoma. If medical therapy fails to control the IOP, glaucoma surgery should be undertaken; the options to consider include aqueous tube shunt, filtering procedure with antimetabolite therapy, or diode laser cyclodestruction.

For eyes with no useful vision, the goal of treatment becomes patient comfort. The options for blind painful eyes that fail to respond to medical therapy include cyclodestruction, retrobulbar alcohol injection, or enucleation.

REFERENCES

1. Hoskins HD Jr, Kass MA. *Becker-Shaffer's Diagnosis and Therapy of the Glaucomas*. 6th ed. St. Louis, Mo: The CV Mosby Company; 1989:253.

2. Maumenee AE, Paton D, Morse PH, Butner P. Review of 40 histologically proven cases of epithelial downgrowth following cataract extraction and suggested surgical management. *Am J Ophthalmol*. 1970;69:598-603.

3. Weiner MJ, Trentacoste J, Pon DM, Albert DM. Epithelial downgrowth: a 30-year clinicopathological review. *Br J Ophthalmol*. 1989;73:6-11.

4. Luntz MH. Glaucoma associated with uveitis (hypertensive glaucoma). In: El Sayad F, Spaeth GL, Shields MB, Hitchings RA, eds. *The Refractory Glaucomas*. Tokyo, Japan: Igaku-Shoin; 1995:91-106.

5. Bill A. Editorial: The drainage of aqueous humor. *Invest Ophthalmol*. 1975;14:1-3.

6. Ritch R. Pathophysiology of glaucoma in uveitis. *Trans Ophthalmol Soc UK*. 1981;101:321-324.

17

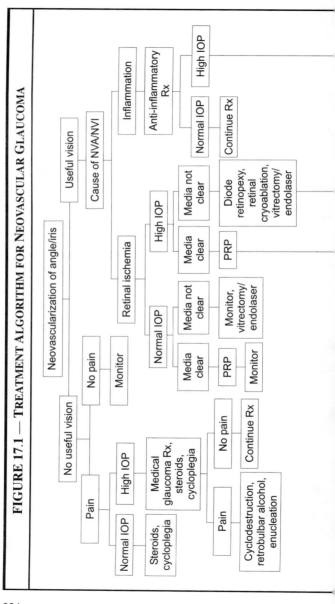

FIGURE 17.1 — TREATMENT ALGORITHM FOR NEOVASCULAR GLAUCOMA

- Medical glaucoma Rx
- Glaucoma surgery:
  - Trabeculectomy with antimetabolite
  - Aqueous tube shunt
  - Diode laser cyclophotocoagulation

Abbreviations: IOP, intraocular pressure; NVA/NVI, neovascularization of angle/iris; PRP, panretinal photocoagulation; Rx, therapy.

Adapted from: Sivak-Callcott JA, et al. *Ophthalmology*. 2001;108:1767-1776.

17

7.   Wilhelminus KR, Grierson I, Watson PG. Factors in the etiology of secondary glaucoma. *Am J Ophthalmol.* 1981;91:697.

8.   Watson PG, Hayreh SS. Scleritis and episcleritis. *Br J Ophthalmol.* 1976;60:163-191.

9.   Goldberg I. Ocular inflammatory and corticosteroid-induced glaucoma. In: Yanoff M, Duker JS, eds. *Ophthalmology.* London: Mosby; 1999:12.17.1-6.

10.   American Academy of Ophthalmology. *Glaucoma. Basic and Clinical Science Course 2003-2004.* San Francisco, Calif: American Academy of Ophthalmology; 2003:89.

11.   Hogan MJ, Kimura ST, Thygeson P. Pathology of herpes simplex kerato-iritis. *Am J Ophthalmol.* 1964;57:551.

12.   Falcon MG, Williams HP. Herpes simplex kerato-uveitis and glaucoma. *Trans Ophthalmol Soc UK.* 1978;98:101-104.

13.   Womack LW, Liesegang TJ. Complications of herpes zoster ophthalmicus. *Arch Ophthalmol.* 1983;101:42-45.

14.   Sundmacher R, Neumann-Haefelin D. Herpes simplex virus isolation from the aqueous of patients suffering from focal iritis, endotheliitis, and prolonged discoform keratitis with glaucoma. *Klin Monatsbl Augenheikd.* 1979;175:488-501.

15.   McGill J, Chapman C. A comparison of topical acyclovir with steroids in the treatment of herpes zoster keratouveitis. *Br J Ophthalmol.* 1983;67:746-750.

16.   Mermoud A, Heuer DK. Glaucoma associated with trauma. In: Ritch R, Shields MB, Krupin T, eds. *The Glaucomas.* 2nd ed. St. Louis, Mo: Mosby; 1996:1259-1275.

17.   Barton K. Secondary glaucomas: classification and management. In: Hitchings RA, ed. *Glaucoma.* London: BMJ Publishing Group; 2000:196-213.

18.   Berke SJ. Post-traumatic glaucoma. In: Yanoff M, Duker JS, eds. *Ophthalmology.* London: Mosby; 1999:12.18.1-4.

19.   Kaufman JH, Tolpin DW. Glaucoma after traumatic angle recession. A ten-year prospective study. *Am J Ophthalmol.* 1974;78:648-654.

20. Edwards WC, Layden WE. Traumatic hyphema. A report of 184 consecutive cases. *Am J Ophthalmol.* 1973;75:110-116.

21. Volpe NJ, Larrison WI, Hersh PS, Kim T, Shingleton BJ. Secondary hemorrhage in traumatic hyphema. *Am J Ophthalmol.* 1991;112:507-513.

22. Spaeth GL, Levy PM. Traumatic hyphema: its clinical characteristics and failure of estrogens to alter it course. A double-blind study. *Am J Ophthalmol.* 1966;62:1098-1106.

23. Sivak-Callcott JA, O'Day DM, Gass JD, Tsai JC. Evidence-based recommendations for the diagnosis and treatment of neovascular glaucoma. *Ophthalmology.* 2001;108:1767-1776.

17

INDEX

Note: Page numbers in *italics* indicate figures;
page numbers followed by t refer to tables.

18

18

18

233

18

235

18

18

239

18

243

18

18

18

252